RSA00000

ISBN #0-9679546-1-4

Cellular Health Series:

The Heart

Matthias Rath, M.D.

First Edition, February 2001

TABLE OF CONTENTS

1 **Introduction** 9

21st Century - Eradicating Heart Disease
10 - Step Program to Optimum Cardiovascular Health
Biological Fuel For Millions of Cardiovascular Cells
Cellular Health

2 **Atherosclerosis, Heart Attack and Stroke** 25

The Facts About Coronary Heart Disease
Vitamins and Other Nutrients Can Halt and Reverse
Coronary Heart Disease
Clinical Studies Document Prevention of Cardiovascular
Disease with Vitamins
Importance of Nutrients for Optimal Cardiovascular Health
The Natural Reversal of Cardiovascular Disease

3 **High Cholesterol Levels and Other** 55
Secondary Risk Factors for Cardiovascular Disease

Cholesterol Is Only a Secondary Risk Factor
How Vitamins Can Help in Normalizing Cholesterol Levels
Clinical Studies with Vitamins Document the Natural
Lowering of Risk Factors In Blood

4 **High Blood Pressure** 71

The Facts About High Blood Pressure
Vitamins in Optimizing Heart Muscle Function
Clinical Evidence that Vitamins and Other Nutrients Can
Optimize Heart Musle Function
Further Clincal Studies with Vitamins
Problems with Incomplete Treatment of Heart Failure

TABLE OF CONTENTS

5 **Heart Failure** **79**

The Facts About Heart Failure
Vitamins in Optimizing Heart Muscle Function
Clinical Evidence that Vitamins and Other Nutrients Can
Optimize Heart Muscle Function
Further Clinical studies with Vitamins
Problems with Incomplete Treatment of Heart Failure

6 **Irregular Heartbeat (Arrhythmia)** **93**

Facts About Irregular Heartbeat
Vitamins in Optimizing Heart Pumping Function
Clinical Studies in Arrhythmia

7 **Diabetes** **101**

The Facts About Vitamins and Adult Diabetes
Cardiovascular Complications in Diabetes
Clinical Studies Document Effectiveness of
Vitamins in Diabetic Conditions

8 **Specific Cardiovascular Problems** **113**

Vitamins and Angina Pectoris
Vitamins After A Heart Attack
Vitamins and Coronary Bypass Surgery
Vitamins and Coronary Angioplasty

TABLE OF CONTENTS

9 External and Inherited CardiovascularRisks   **129**

- Unhealthy Diet
- Smoking
- Stress
- Hormonal Contraceptives
- Diuretic Medication
- Other Prescription Drugs
- Dialysis
- Surgery
- Inherited Cardiovascular Risk Factors

10 Cellular Health and Vitamins   **147**

Vitamins and Other Nutrients As Bioenergy Source
The Goal of Cellular Health
Scientific Facts About the Ingredients of Dr.Rath's
Vitamin Program
Vitamin Programs Compared to Conventional Therapies

11 The Path to Eradicating Heart Disease   **169**

New Era of Human Health Begins
Principles of a New Health Care System
The Rath-Pauling Manifesto
About the Author

Acknowledgments

My thanks go to all those without whom the medical break-through towards control of cardiovascular disease would be delayed by many years.

My thanks also go to all those who have remained an invaluable source of motivation for me through their skepticism and opposition.

Dr. Matthias Rath

Introduction

1

21st Century – Eradicating Heart Disease

10-Step Program To Optimum Cardiovascular Health

Biological Fuel For Millions Of Cardiovascular Cells

Cellular Health

Dr. Rath's challenge to the people of the world:

Only once in the course of human events comes the time when heart attacks, strokes and other cardiovascular conditions can be eradicated. The time is now. Just as the discovery that microorganisms cause infectious diseases led to the control of infectious epidemics so will the discovery that heart attacks and strokes are the result of long-term vitamin deficiencies lead to the control of the cardiovascular epidemic. Mankind can eradicate heart disease as a major cause of death and disability during the 21st century.

Animals don't get heart attacks because they produce vitamin C in their bodies, which protects their blood vessel walls. In humans, who are unable to produce vitamin C, dietary vitamin deficiency weakens these walls. Cardiovascular disease is an early form of scurvy. Clinical studies document that optimum daily intake of vitamins and other essential nutrients halts and reverses coronary heart disease. These essential nutrients supply vital bioenergy to millions of heart and blood vessel cells, thereby optimizing cardiovascular functions. Optimum supply of vitamins and other essential nutrients can prevent and help correct cardiovascular conditions naturally. Heart attacks, strokes, high blood pressure, irregular heartbeat, heart failure, circulatory problems in diabetes, and other cardiovascular problems, will be unknown in future generations.

Eradicating heart disease is the next great goal for mankind to overcome. The availability of vitamins and other essential nutrients needed to control the global cardiovascular epidemic is unlimited. The eradication of heart disease is dependent on one single factor: How quickly we can spread the message that vitamins and other essential nutrients are the solution to the cardiovascular epidemic.

Let's eradicate heart disease during this century!

The last decade of the 20th century was characterized by continuing efforts to block the spread of this life-saving information in order to protect a global prescription drug market. But the will of the people to gain free access to natural health information was stronger than the interests defending the "Business with Disease."

We, the people of the world, must recognize that our combined effort has created the opportunity to eradicate cardiovascular disease and other diseases that are caused largely by chronic vitamin deficiencies.

- **We proclaim the 21st Century the "Century of Eradicating Heart Disease."**

- **We will spread information about the life-saving benefits of vitamins.**

- **We now call for a new health care system.**

A hundred years ago: Eradicating epidemics

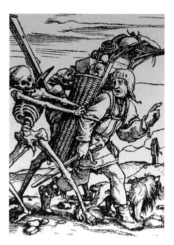

For millennia, infectious diseases were the number one cause of death, and billions of people died from them.

For millennia people believed that the cause of these epidemics was a curse of heaven.

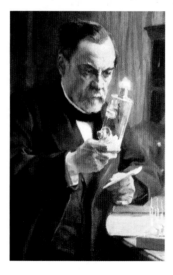

Then 150 years ago Louis Pasteur discovered that these epidemics were caused by bacteria and other microorganisms.

This discovery enabled the implementation of preventive methods, as well as the development of vaccines and antibiotics.

A few years ago, the World Health Organization (WHO) declared smallpox the first infectious disease to be eradicated.

Today: Eradicating heart disease

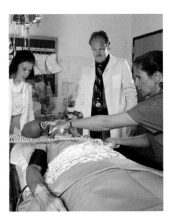

During the 20th century, cardiovascular diseases became the number one cause of death in the industrialized world. Over a billion people have died worldwide during the last century from heart attacks and strokes.

Because the main cause of cardiovascular disease has remained unknown until now, the cardiovascular epidemic continues to spread on a global scale.

This book documents the solution to the cardiovascular epidemic: Animals don't get heart attacks because – as opposed to humans – they produce vitamin C in their bodies. Heart attacks and strokes are not diseases but the consequence of chronic vitamin deficiency and they are, therefore, preventable.

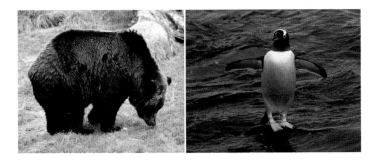

13

Dr. Rath's 10-Step Program for Optimum Cardiovascular Health

The medical breakthrough documented in this book can be summarized in a practical 10-step-program of essential nutrients:

1 Be aware of the size and function of your cardiovascular system.

Did you know that your blood vessel pipeline system measures 60,000 miles and is the largest organ in your body? Optimizing your cardiovascular health benefits your entire body and your overall health. Because your body is as old as your cardiovascular system, optimizing your cardiovascular health adds years to your life.

2 Stabilize the walls of your blood vessels.

Blood vessel instability and lesions in your blood vessel walls are the primary causes for cardiovascular disease. Vitamin C is the cement of the blood vessel walls and stabilizes them. Animals don't get heart disease because they produce enough endogenous vitamin C in their livers to protect their blood vessels. In contrast, humans develop deposits leading to heart attacks and strokes because we cannot manufacture our own vitamin C and generally get too few vitamins in our diet.

3 Reverse artery deposits naturally without surgery.

Cholesterol and fat particles are deposited inside the blood vessel walls by means of biological adhesives. "Teflon"-like agents can prevent this stickiness. The amino acids, lysine and proline are Nature's "Teflon" agents. Together with vitamin C, they help reverse existing deposits naturally.

4 Relax your blood vessel walls.

Deposits and spasms of the blood vessel walls are the causes of high blood pressure. Dietary supplementation of magnesium, arginine and vitamin C relaxes the blood vessel walls and helps normalize high blood pressure.

5 Optimize the performance of your heart.

The heart is the motor of the cardiovascular system. Like the motor of your car, millions of muscle cells need cell fuel for optimum performance. Nature's cell fuels include carnitine, coenzyme Q-10, B vitamins, and many other nutrients and trace elements. Dietary supplementation of these essential nutrients will optimize the performance of the heart and contribute to a regular heartbeat.

6 Protect your cardiovascular pipelines from rusting.
Biological rusting, or oxidation, damages your cardiovascular system and accelerates the aging process. Vitamin C, vitamin E, beta-carotene, and selenium are the most important natural antioxidants. Other important antioxidants are bioflavonoids, such as pycnogenol. Dietary supplementation of these antioxidants provides important rust protection for your cardiovascular system. Above all, stop smoking because cigarette smoke accelerates the biological rusting of your blood vessels.

7 Exercise regularly.
Regular physical activity is an important step for optimum cardio-vascular health. Regular exercise, like walking or bicycling, is ideal and can be performed by everybody.

8 Eat a prudent diet.
The diet of our ancestors over thousands of generations was rich in plant nutrition and high in fiber and vitamins. These dietary preferences shaped the metabolism of our bodies today. A diet rich in fruits and vegetables and low in fat and sugars enhances your cardiovascular health.

9 Find time to relax.
Physical and emotional stresses are cardiovascular risk factors. Schedule hours and days to relax as you would schedule your appointments. Moreover, the production of the stress hormone adrenaline requires vitamin C. Long-term physical or emotional stress depletes your body's vitamin pool and requires dietary vita-min supplementation.

10 Start now.
Thickening of the blood vessel walls is not only a problem of the elderly, it starts in your twenties. Early intervention equals active protection of your cardiovascular system.

Biological Fuel For Millions of Cardiovascular Cells

Throughout this book you will read about the remarkable health effects of vitamins and other essential nutrients. The scientific basis of these dramatic health improvements can be summarized as follows: the cells in our body fulfill a multitude of functions. Gland cells produce hormones; white blood cells produce antibodies; heart muscle cells generate and conduct biological electricity for the heartbeat. The specific function of each cell is determined by the genetic software program, the genes located in each cell core.

Despite these different functions, the same carriers of bioenergy and the same biocatalysts produce a multitude of biochemical reactions inside all cells. Many of these essential biocatalysts and bioenergy molecules cannot be produced by the body itself and have to be supplemented in our diet on a regular basis. Vitamins, certain amino acids, minerals, and trace elements are among the most important essential nutrients for optimum function of each cell. Without optimum intake of these essential nutrients, the function of millions of cells becomes impaired and diseases develop.

Unfortunately, conventional medicine fails to recognize the decisive role of vitamins and other essential nutrients for optimum cellular function and for optimum health. The modern concept of Cellular Health will fundamentally change that. In a few years, daily supplementation with vitamins, minerals and other essential nutrients will be a matter of course for everyone, just like eating and drinking.

Single cell (schematic)

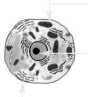

Cellular Power Plant
(Mitochondrium)

Cellular Core
Central Unit
(Nucleus)

Cellular Production Line
(Endoplasmic Reticulum)

Important Biocatalysts:

- Vitamin C
- Vitamin B-1
- Vitamin B-3
- Vitamin B-5
- Vitamin B-6
- Vitamin B-12

- Carnitine
- Coenzyme Q-10
- Minerals
- Trace elements

The metabolic software program of each cell is determined by the genetic information in each cell core. Essential nutrients are needed as biocatalysts and as carriers of bioenergy in each cell. Both functions are essential for optimum performance of millions of cells.

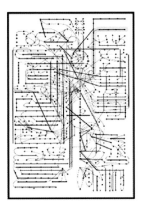

Cellular Health:
The Solution to Optimum Health

The most profound impact of Cellular Health will be in the area of cardiovascular health because this is the most active organ system of our body and therefore has the highest consumption of essential nutrients. The opposite page illustrates the most important cells of the cardiovascular system.

Cells of the blood vessel walls: The endothelial cells form the barrier, or protective layer, between the blood and the blood vessel wall; moreover, these cells contribute to a variety of metabolic functions, such as optimum blood viscosity. The smooth muscle cells produce collagen and other reinforcement molecules, providing optimum stability and tone to the blood vessel walls.

The cells of the heart muscle: The main role of heart muscle cells is the pumping function to maintain blood circulation. A subtype of heart muscle cell is specialized and capable of generating and conducting biological electricity for the heartbeat.

The blood cells: Even the millions of blood corpuscles circulating in the bloodstream are nothing other than cells. They are responsible for transport of oxygen, defense, scavenging, healing, and many other functions. The following pages describe how deficiencies in vitamins and other essential nutrients in these different cell types are closely associated with the most frequent cardiovascular diseases today.

Blood Vessel Wall Cells

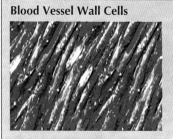 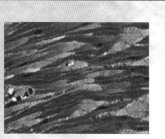

BARRIER CELLS (ENDOTHELIUM)   *VESSEL WALL MUSCLE CELLS*

Blood Cells

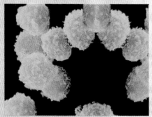 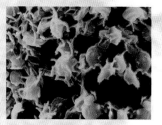

WHITE BLOOD CELLS   *PLATELETS*

Heart Muscle Cells

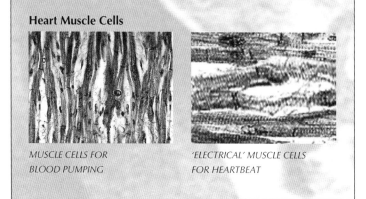

MUSCLE CELLS FOR   *'ELECTRICAL' MUSCLE CELLS*
BLOOD PUMPING   *FOR HEARTBEAT*

THE CARDIOVASCULAR SYSTEM IS COMPOSED OF MILLIONS OF CELLS

Vitamin Deficiency in Artery Wall Cells Causes Heart Attacks, Strokes, and High Blood Pressure

Long-term deficiency of vitamins and other essential nutrients in millions of vascular wall cells impairs the function of the blood vessel walls. The most frequent consequences are high blood pressure conditions and the development of atherosclerotic deposits which lead to heart attacks and strokes.

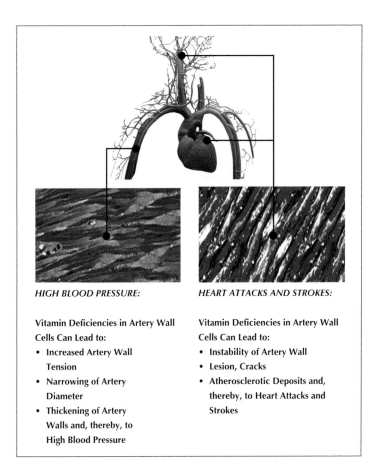

HIGH BLOOD PRESSURE:

Vitamin Deficiencies in Artery Wall Cells Can Lead to:
- **Increased Artery Wall Tension**
- **Narrowing of Artery Diameter**
- **Thickening of Artery Walls and, thereby, to High Blood Pressure**

HEART ATTACKS AND STROKES:

Vitamin Deficiencies in Artery Wall Cells Can Lead to:
- **Instability of Artery Wall**
- **Lesion, Cracks**
- **Atherosclerotic Deposits and, thereby, to Heart Attacks and Strokes**

Vitamin Deficiency in Heart Muscle Cells Causes Irregular Heartbeat and Heart Failure

A chronic deficiency of vitamins and other essential nutrients in millions of heart muscle cells can contribute to an impaired heart function. The most frequent consequences are irregular heartbeat (arrhythmia) and heart failure (shortness of breath, edema, and fatigue).

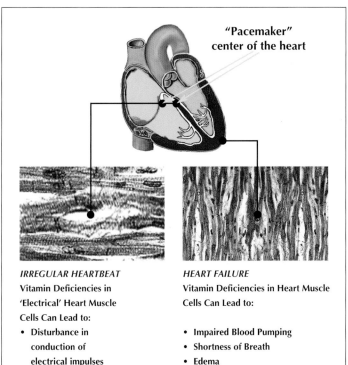

"Pacemaker" center of the heart

IRREGULAR HEARTBEAT
Vitamin Deficiencies in 'Electrical' Heart Muscle Cells Can Lead to:
- Disturbance in conduction of electrical impulses for the heartbeat

- Irregular Heartbeat

HEART FAILURE
Vitamin Deficiencies in Heart Muscle Cells Can Lead to:

- Impaired Blood Pumping
- Shortness of Breath
- Edema
- Severe Fatigue

Notes

2

Atherosclerosis, Heart Attack and Stroke

The Facts About Coronary Heart Disease

Vitamins and other Nutrients Can Halt and Reverse Coronary Heart Disease

Clinical Studies Document Prevention Of Cardiovascular Disease With Vitamins

Importance of Nutrients for Optimal Cardiovascular Health

The Natural Reversal of Cardiovascular Disease

The Facts About Coronary Heart Disease

- **Every year, every other death** in the industrialized world is due to atherosclerotic deposits in the coronary arteries (leading to heart attack) or in the arteries supplying blood to the brain (leading to stroke). The epidemic spread of these cardiovascular diseases is largely due to the fact that until now the true nature of atherosclerosis and coronary heart disease has not been understood.

- **Conventional medicine** is largely confined to treating the symptoms of this disease. Calcium antagonists, beta-blockers, nitrates, and other drugs are prescribed to alleviate angina pain. Surgical procedures (angioplasty, bypass surgery) are applied to improve blood flow mechanically. Hardly any conventional medicine targets the underlying problem: the instability of the vascular wall which triggers the development of atherosclerotic deposits.

- **Cellular Health** provides a breakthrough in our understanding of these causes and leads to effective prevention and treatment of coronary heart disease. The primary cause of coronary heart disease and other forms of atherosclerotic disease is a chronic deficiency of vitamins and other essential nutrients in millions of vascular wall cells. This leads to instability of the vascular walls, to lesions and cracks, to atherosclerotic deposits, and eventually to heart attacks or strokes. Since the primary cause of cardiovascular disease is a deficiency of essential nutrients in the vascular wall, a daily optimum intake of these essential nutrients is the primary measure to prevent atherosclerosis and to help repair vascular wall damage.

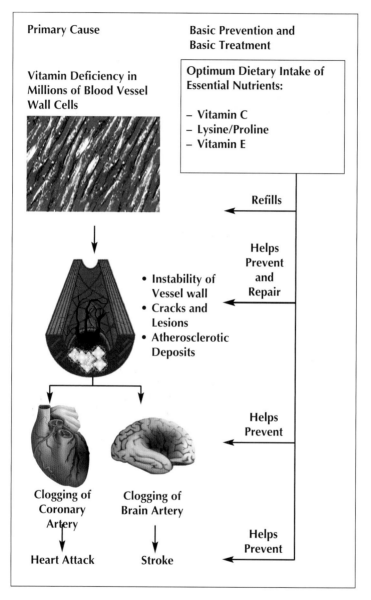

CORONARY ARTERY DISEASE AND OTHER FORMS OF ATHEROSCLEROTIC CARDIOVASCULAR DISEASE

Vitamins and Other Nutrients Can Halt and Reverse Coronary Heart Disease

Millions of people die every year from heart attacks because no effective treatment to halt or to reverse coronary artery disease has been available. Therefore, we decided to test the efficacy of a defined vitamin program for the Number One health problem of our time: coronary atherosclerosis, the cause of heart attacks. We realized that if this nutritional supplement program could stop further growth of coronary atherosclerosis, the fight against heart attacks could be won and the goal of eradicating heart disease would become reality.

To measure the success of this vitamin program we focused on the key problem, the atherosclerotic deposits inside the walls of the coronary arteries. A fascinating new diagnostic technique had just become available that allowed us to measure the size of the coronary deposits non-invasively: Ultrafast Computed Tomography.

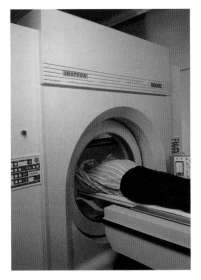

Ultrafast CT, the "mammogram of the heart," is a new diagnostic technology that allows non-invasive testing for coronary artery disease.

The Ultrafast CT measures areas and density of the calcium deposits without any needles or radioactive dye; then the computer automatically calculates their size by determining the Coronary Artery Scan (CAS) score. The higher the CAS score, the more calcium has accumulated, indicating more advanced coronary artery disease. Compared to angiography and treadmill tests, Ultrafast CT is the most precise diagnostic technique available today to detect coronary artery disease. This diagnostic test finds deposits in coronary arteries long before a patient notices any symptoms.

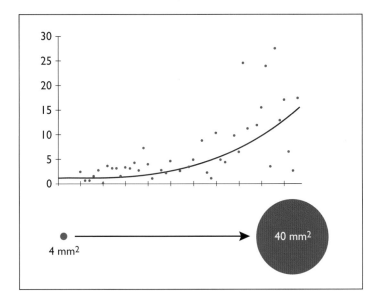

Growth Rate of Coronary Deposits Per Year in Each Patient
Without vitamins, the atherosclerotic plaques in the coronary arteries increased exponentially. This picture shows the growth rate of coronary deposits in each patient before the vitamin program started. Patients with early coronary artery disease had an average increase of plaque area of 4 mm^2 every year (left side of the figure). The deposits of patients with advanced coronary artery disease increased by 40 mm^2 and more every year (right side).

Moreover, since it directly measures the deposits in the artery walls, it is a much better indicator for a person's cardiovascular risk than any measurements of cholesterol or other risk factors in the bloodstream.

We studied 55 patients with various degrees of coronary artery disease. Changes in the size of the coronary artery calcifications in each patient were measured over an average period of one year without the vitamin program, followed by a period of one year with the vitamin program. In this way, the heart scans of the same person could be compared. This study design had the advantage that the patients served as their own controls. All of the essential nutrients given in this program have a synergistic effect.

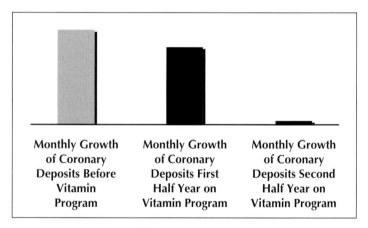

Synergistic Action of Nutrients Can Stop Coronary Heart Disease Before You Even Feel It.
With vitamin programs the fast growth of coronary artery deposits can be slowed down during the first half year and essentially stopped within the second half year. Thus, no heart attacks will develop. These are the study results from patients with early coronary deposits, who, like millions of adults in the prime of their lives, developed heart disease without feeling it.

The results of this landmark study were published in the Journal of Applied Nutrition in 1996 (see reference listing at the end of this book). The most important findings are also presented here. This study measured how aggressively coronary artery disease grows until a heart attack occurs. Without supplement intake, the coronary calcifications increased at an exponential rate, with an average growth of 44% every year. Thus, without vitamin protection, coronary deposits add about half their size every year.

When patients started the vitamin program, this trend was reversed and the average growth rate of coronary calcifications actually slowed. Most significantly, in patients with early stages of coronary heart disease, this essential nutrient program stopped further growth of coronary heart disease within one year. Thus, this study also gives us valuable information about the time nutrients take until they show their healing effect on the artery wall. While for the first six months the deposits in these patients continued to grow at a decreased pace, the growth essentially stops during the second six months on this vitamin program. Of course, any therapy that stops coronary artery disease in its early stages prevents heart attacks later.

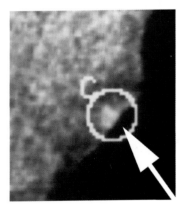 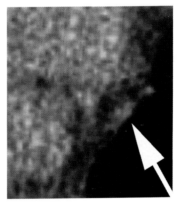

Before   **After**

NATURAL HEALING OF CORONARY ARTERY DISEASE
Before the vitamin program the patient had developed atherosclerotic deposits in the walls of his left coronary artery (white circled area in the left picture). The above pictures are magnifications from the heart scan X-ray pictures taken with the computer tomograph.

It is not surprising that several months pass until the healing effect of vitamins and other nutrients on the artery wall becomes noticeable. Atherosclerotic deposits develop over many years or decades, and it takes several months to control this aggressive disease and start the healing process. More advanced stages of coronary heart disease may take longer before the vascular healing process is measurable.

Breakthrough in Natural Health

This clinical study marks a major breakthrough in medicine and will lead to health improvements for millions of people throughout the world. For the first time, the following clinical results were documented:

- Without vitamin therapy, coronary artery disease is a very aggressive disease and the deposits grow on average at a staggering rate of 44% per year.
- Vitamins and other nutrients are able to halt coronary atherosclerosis, the cause of heart attacks, in its early stages.
- Thus, there now exists an effective natural approach to prevent, and to reverse, coronary heart disease naturally – without angioplasty or bypass surgery.
- Every person anywhere in the world can immediately take advantage of this medical breakthrough.
- During the next decades, deaths from heart attacks and strokes will be reduced to a fraction of their current toll, and cardiovascular disease will essentially be unknown to future generations.

Large-Scale Studies Document Prevention of Cardiovascular Disease With Vitamins

The importance of various vitamins and other nutrients in the prevention of cardiovascular disease has also been documented in numerous clinical and epidemiological studies.

Dr. James Enstrom and his colleagues from the University of California in Los Angeles investigated vitamin intake of more than 11,000 Americans over ten years. This government-supported study showed that people who took at least 300 mg per day of vitamin C, compared to 50 mg contained in an average American diet, could reduce their heart disease rate up to 50% in men and up to 40% in women. The same study showed that an increased intake of vitamin C was associated with an increased life expectancy of up to six years.

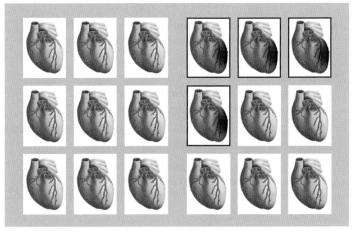

300 mg Vitamin C per Day: *Average Diet*:
Up to 50% Fewer Heart Attacks   **Increased Risk for Heart Attacks**

Vitamin C Cuts Risk for Heart Attacks in Half

The Canadian physician, Dr. G. C. Willis, showed that dietary vitamin C can reverse atherosclerosis. At the beginning of his study, he documented the atherosclerotic deposits in his patients by angiography (injection of a radioactive substance followed by X-ray pictures). After this documentation, half of the patients received 1.5 grams of vitamin C per day. The other half of the patients received no additional vitamin C. The control analysis, on average, after 10 to 12 months, showed that in those patients who received additional vitamin C, the atherosclerotic deposits decreased in 30% of the cases. In contrast, no decrease in atherosclerotic deposits could be seen in those patients without vitamin C supplementation. The deposits in these patients either remained the same or had further increased. Amazingly, this important clinical study was conducted more than 40 years ago.

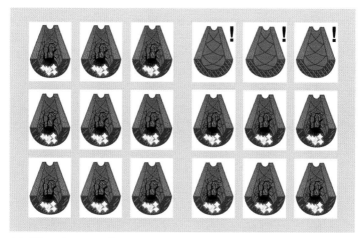

No Vitamin C Supplements:
Coronary Deposits grow

1500 mg Vitamin C per Day:
Halt and reversal in 30% of the cases

Vitamin C Cuts Risk for Heart Attacks in Half

35

Vitamin E and Beta Carotene Also Decrease Your Cardiovascular Risk

The Nurses' Health Study included more than 87,000 American nurses, ages 34 to 59. In 1993, the first result was published in the New England Journal of Medicine. It was shown that study participants taking more than 200 units of vitamin E per day could reduce their risk for heart attacks by 34%, compared to those receiving only 3 units, the average daily intake of vitamin E in Americans.

The Health Professional Study included over 39,000 health professionals, ages 40 to 75. At the beginning of the study, none of the participants had any signs of cardiovascular disease or diabetes, or elevated blood cholesterol levels. The study showed that people taking 400 units of vitamin E per day could reduce their risk for heart attack by 40%, compared to those taking only 6 units of vitamin E per day.

The Physicians Health Study included over 22,000 physicians, ages 40 to 84. From this study in patients with existing cardiovascular disease, published by Dr. Hennekens in 1992, it was shown that in those patients, 50 mg of beta carotene per day could cut the risk for suffering a heart attack or stroke in half.

- Vitamin C intake lowers cardiovascular risk by 50%, documented in 11,000 study participants over 10 years.

- Vitamin E supplementation lowers cardiovascular risk by one-third, documented in 87,000 study participants over 6 years.

- Beta carotene supplementation lowers cardiovascular risk by over 50%, documented in more than 22,000 study participants.

- No prescription drug has ever been shown to be as effective as these vitamins in preventing heart disease.

Important Nutrients for Optimum Cardiovascular Health

The following cellular bioenergy factors are important to optimize the function of cells that build blood vessel walls and the heart muscle. They should be part of your dietary program in addition to a healthy diet.

- **Vitamin C:** protection and natural healing of the artery wall, reversal of plaques.

- **Vitamin E:** anti-oxidant protection.

- **Vitamin D:** optimizing of calcium metabolism, reversal of calcium deposits in artery walls.

- **Proline:** collagen production, stability of the artery wall, reversal of plaques.

- **Lysine:** collagen production, stability of the artery wall, reversal of plaques.

- **Folic acid:** protective function against increased homo-cysteine levels together with Vitamin B6, Vitamin B12 and Biotin.

- **Biotin:** protective function against increased homocys-teine levels together with Vitamin B6, Vitamin B12 and folic acid.

- **Copper:** stability of the artery wall by improved cross-linking of collagen molecules.

- **Chondroitin sulfate:** stability of the artery wall as "cement" of the artery wall connective tissue.

- **N-Acetylglycosamine:** stability of the artery wall as "cement" of the artery wall connective tissue.

- **Pycnogenol:** biocatalyst for improved vitamin C function, improved stability of the artery walls.

Importance of Nutrients for Optimal Cardiovascular Health

What Is Atherosclerosis?

The pictures on this page are cross-sections from arteries of patients with coronary artery disease. The dark ring you notice is the original blood vessel wall as it would be found in a newborn baby. The pink area within this dark ring is athero-sclerotic deposits which developed over many years.

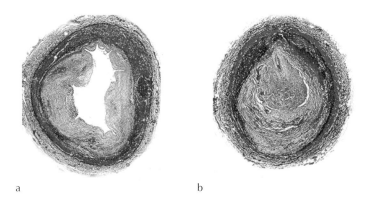

a   b

Picture A shows atherosclerotic deposits in coronary arteries, which reduce blood flow and impair oxygen and nutrient supply to millions of heart muscle cells. The coronary arteries of patients with angina pectoris typically look like this.

Picture B shows the coronary arteries of a patient who died from a heart attack. On top of the atherosclerotic deposits, a blood clot formed that completely interrupted the blood flow through this artery. This is called a heart attack. Millions of heart muscle cells die, leaving the heart muscle permanently impaired or leading to the death of the patient.

It is important to understand that the atherosclerotic deposits in Picture A have developed over many years. In contrast, the additional blood clot in Picture B develops within minutes or seconds. Effective prevention of heart attacks has to start as early as possible by preventing atherosclerotic deposits. Atherosclerosis is not a disease of advanced age. Studies of soldiers killed in the Korean and Vietnam wars showed that up to 75% of the victims had already developed some form of atherosclerotic deposits at age 25 and younger. The picture below shows a coronary artery of a 25-year-old victim of a traffic accident. This coincidental finding shows how far atherosclerosis can advance in young adults – without causing any symptoms.

The main cause of atherosclerotic deposits is the biological weakness of the artery walls caused by chronic vitamin deficiency. The atherosclerotic deposits are the consequence of this chronic weakness; they develop as a compensatory stabilizing cast to strengthen these weakened blood vessel walls.

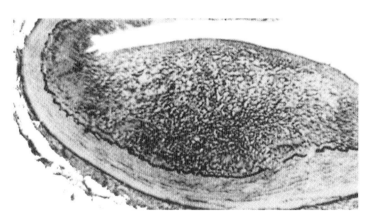

CROSS SECTION (MAGNIFIED) OF THE CORONARY ARTERY OF A 25-YEAR-OLD VICTIM OF A TRAFFIC ACCIDENT. THE ATHEROSCLEROTIC DEPOSITS HAD DEVELOPED WITHOUT THE YOUNG MAN KNOWING OR NOTICING ANYTHING.

Why Animals Don't Get Heart Attacks

According to the statistics of the World Health Organization, each year more than 12,000,000 people die from of heart attacks and strokes. Amazingly, while cardiovascular disease has become one of the largest epidemics ever to haunt mankind, these very same heart attacks are unknown in the animal world. The following paragraph from the renowned textbook of veterinary medicine by Professor H. A. Smith and T. C. Jones documents these facts:

> "The fact remains, however, that in none of the domestic species, with the rarest of exceptions, do animals develop atherosclerotic disease of clinical significance. It appears that most of the pertinent pathological mechanisms operate in animals and that atherosclerotic disease in them is not impossible; **it just does not occur.** If the reason for this could be found it might cast some very useful light on the human disease."

These important observations were published in 1958. Now, over four decades later, the puzzle of human cardiovascular disease has been solved. The solution to the puzzle of human cardiovascular disease is one of the great advances in medicine.

Here is the main reason why animals don't get heart attacks: With few exceptions, animals produce vitamin C in their bodies. The daily amounts of vitamin C produced vary between 1000 mg and 20,000 mg, when compared to the human body weight. Vitamin C is the cement of the artery wall, and optimum amounts of vitamin C stabilize the arteries. In contrast, human beings cannot produce a single molecule of vitamin C. Our ancestors lost this ability generations ago when an enzyme that was needed to convert sugar molecules (glucose) into vitamin C became defunct. This change in the molecules of our ancestors had no immediate disadvantage since, for thousands of generations, they relied primarily on

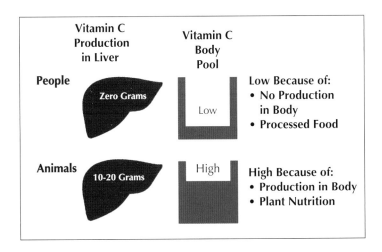

plant nutrition such as cereals, vegetables, and fruit, Nutritional habits and dietary intake of vitamins have changed considerably in this century. Today most people do not receive sufficient amounts of vitamins in their diet. To make matters worse, food processing, long-term storage and overcooking destroy most vitamins in the food. The consequences are summarized in the picture above.

The single most important difference between the metabolism of human beings and most other living species is the dramatic difference in the body pool of vitamin C. The body reservoir of vitamin C in people is on average ten to 100 times lower than the vitamin C levels in animals.

How Does Vitamin C Prevent Atherosclerosis?

Vitamin C contributes to the prevention of cardiovascular disease in many different ways. It is an important antioxidant, and it serves as a cofactor for many biochemical reactions in the body cells. The most important function of vitamin C in preventing heart attacks and strokes is its ability to increase the production of collagen, elastin, and other reinforcement molecules in the body. These biological reinforcement rods

41

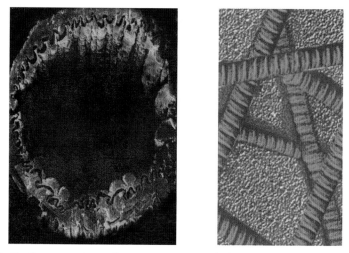

Left: *Cross section of an artery (magnified).Collagen and other connnective tissue (white structures) provide basic stability to blood vessel walls.*

Right: *Individual collagen molecules under high magnification. Each of these fibers is stronger than a metal wire of comparable width.*

constitute the connective tissue, about 50% of all proteins in our body. Collagen has the same function for our body as iron reinforcement rods have for a skyscraper building. Increased production of collagen means improved stability for the 60,000-mile-long walls of our arteries, veins, and capillaries.

The Scientific World Knows The Facts

The close connection between vitamin C deficiency and the instability of body tissue was established long ago. The following page is taken from the world-famous textbook on biochemistry by Professor Lubert Stryer of Stanford University.

Scurvy Is Caused by Collagen Deficiency

The importance of the hydroxylation of collagen becomes evident in scurvy. A vivid description of this disease was given by Jacques Cartier in 1536, when it afflicted his men as they were exploring the Saint Lawrence River:

"Some did lose all their strength and could not stand on their feet...others also had all their skins spotted with spots of blood of a purple color: then did it ascend up to their ankles, knees, thighs, shoulders, arms and necks. Their mouths became stinking, their gums so rotten, that all the flesh did fall off, even to the roots of the teeth which did also almost all fall out."

The means of preventing scurvy was succinctly stated by James Lind, a Scottish physician, in 1753: "Experience indeed sufficiently shows that as greens or fresh vegetables with ripe fruits, are the best remedies for it, so they prove the most effectual preservatives against it." Lind urged the inclusion of lemon juice in the diet of sailors. His advice was adopted by the British navy some 40 years later.

Scurvy is caused by a dietary deficiency of ascorbic acid (vitamin C). Primates and guinea pigs have lost the ability to synthesize ascorbic acid and so they must acquire it from their diets. Ascorbic acid, an effective reducing agent, maintains prolyl hydroxylase in an active form, probably by keeping its iron atom in the reduced ferrous state. Collagen synthesized in the absence of ascorbic acid is insufficiently hydroxylated and, hence, has a lower melting temperature. This abnormal collagen cannot properly form fibers and thus causes the skin lesions and blood vessel fragility that are so prominent in scurvy.

Atherosclerosis Is An Early Form Of Scurvy

While these facts were known 250 years ago, they are still not applied in medicine today. The next figure summarizes the fact that the main cause of heart attacks and strokes is a scurvy-like condition of the artery wall.

Left column A: Optimum intake of vitamin C leads to an optimum production and function of collagen molecules. A stable blood vessel wall does not allow atherosclerotic deposits to develop. Optimum availability of vitamin C in their bodies is the main reason why animals don't get heart attacks.

Center column B: Atherosclerosis and cardiovascular disease are exactly between these two conditions. Our average diet contains enough vitamin C to prevent open scurvy, but not enough to guarantee stable reinforced artery walls. As a consequence, millions of tiny cracks and lesions develop along the artery walls. Subsequently, cholesterol, lipoproteins, and other blood risk factors enter the damaged artery walls in order to repair these lesions. With chronic low vitamin intake, however, this repair process continues over decades. Over many years this repair overcompensates or overshoots and atherosclerotic deposits develop. Deposits in the arteries of the heart eventually lead to heart attack; deposits in the arteries of the brain lead to stroke..

Right column C: The right column of this figure summarizes the events in scurvy. Total depletion of the vitamin C body reserves, as they occurred in sailors of earlier centuries, leads to a gradual break-down of the body's connective tissue, including the vessel walls. Thousands of sailors died within a few months from hemorrhagic blood loss through leaky blood vessel walls.

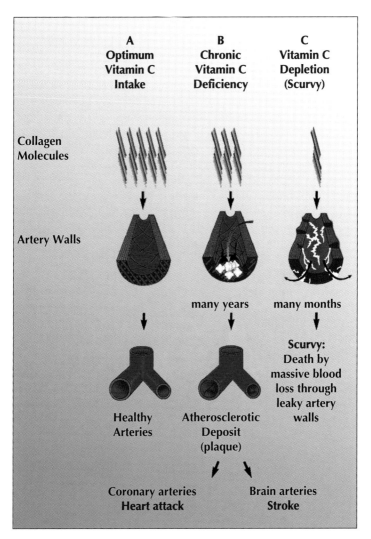

THE SCURVY-CARDIOVASCULAR DISEASE CONNECTION
The connection between cardiovascular disease, vitamin C deficiency, and scurvy is of such fundamental importance for our health that this figure should become an essential part of health education in schools throughout the world.

Vitamin C Deficiency Causes Atherosclerosis - The Proof

It is possible to prove that a deficient intake of vitamin C, without any other factors involved, directly causes atherosclerosis and cardiovascular disease. To prove this, we conducted an animal experiment with guinea pigs, exceptions in the animal world because they share with humans the inability to produce their own vitamin C. Two groups of guinea pigs received exactly the same daily diet, with one exception – vitamin C. Group B received 60 mg of vitamin C per day, compared to the human body weight. This amount was chosen to meet the official recommended daily allowance for humans in the U.S. In contrast, group A received 5,000 mg of vitamin C per day compared to human body weight.

These pictures document the changes in the artery walls in these two groups after only five weeks. The top pictures show the differences in the arteries of the two groups.The vitamin C deficient animals of Group B developed atherosclerotic deposits (white areas), particularly in the areas close to the heart (right side of picture). The aortas of the animals in Group A remained healthy and did not show any deposits. The bottom pictures show the same artery walls examined under a microscope. The artery sections from animals with high vitamin C intake (a) show an intact cell barrier between the bloodstream and the artery wall. The almost parallel alignment of the collagen molecules in the artery wall makes stability visible. In contrast, the arteries of the vitamin C deficient animals (b) have lost the protection (defective barrier cell lining) and stability (fragmented collagen structure) of their arteries. For comparison, a picture of the coronary arteries from a patient with coronary artery disease was added (c).

Note: In principle animal experiments should be kept to an absolute minimum. They are only justified when human lives can be saved with the knowledge that results from these experiments. This was the case with the experiment described, which brought millions of people proof of the value of vitamin C for the prevention of heart attacks.

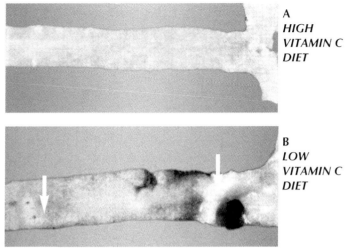

A
*HIGH
VITAMIN C
DIET*

B
*LOW
VITAMIN C
DIET*

THE MAIN ARTERIES (AORTAS) OF ANIMALS ON A HIGH VITAMIN C DIET (TOP PICTURE) AND ON A LOW VITAMIN C DIET (BOTTOM PICTURE). THE WHITE AREAS IN THE BOTTOM PICTURE ARE ATHEROSCLEROTIC DEPOSITS. THESE DEPOSITS ARE NOT THE RESULT OF A HIGH FAT DIET, BUT OF THE BODY'S RESPONSE TO WEAK VITAMIN-DEFICIENT ARTERIES.

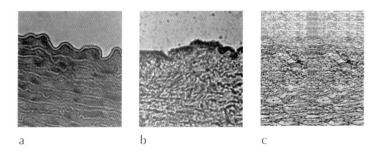

a   b   c

A LOOK INSIDE THREE DIFFERENT ARTERY WALLS UNDER THE MICROSCOPE:
a: Guinea pig on a high vitamin C diet.
b: Guinea pig on a low vitamin C diet.
c: Coronary artery of a patient who had died from a heart attack.

Note the similarity between picture b and c.

A New Understanding of the Nature of Heart Disease

The previous experiment underlines our modern definition of cardiovascular disease as a vitamin deficiency condition. This new understanding is summarized below:

1. **Lesions.** The main cause of cardiovascular disease is the instability and dysfunction of the blood vessel wall caused by chronic vitamin deficiency. This leads to millions of small lesions and cracks in the artery wall, particularly in the coronary arteries. The coronary arteries are the most stressed arteries because they are squeezed flat more than 100,000 times per day, similar to a garden hose which is stepped upon.

2. **Beginning Repair**. Cholesterol and other repair factors are produced at an increased rate in the liver and are transported in the bloodstream to the artery walls, which they enter to mend and repair the damage. Because the coronary arteries sustain the most damage, they require the most intensive repair.

3. **Ongoing Repair**. With continued vitamin deficiency over many years, the repair process in the artery walls overcompensates. (Atherosclerotic plaques form predominantly at those locations in the cardiovascular system with the most intensive repair: the coronary arteries.) This is why infarctions occur primarily at this location and why the most frequent cardiovascular events are infarctions of the heart, not infarctions of the nose or ears.

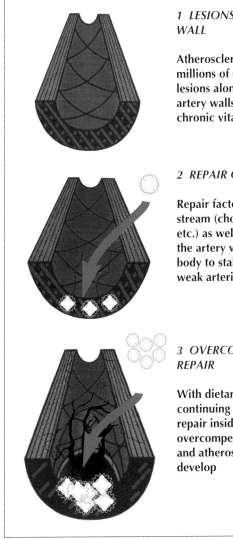

1 LESIONS IN THE ARTERY WALL

Atherosclerosis begins with millions of small cracks and lesions along the inside of the artery walls, as the result of chronic vitamin deficiency

2 REPAIR OF ARTERY WALL

Repair factors from the bloodstream (cholesterol, lipoproteins etc.) as well as cell growth inside the artery walls are used by the body to stabilize and repair the weak arteries

3 OVERCOMPENSATING REPAIR

With dietary vitamin deficiency continuing over many years, this repair inside the artery walls overcompensates or overshoots, and atherosclerotic deposits develop

Atherosclerosis Develops in Three Steps

The Natural Reversal Of Cardiovascular Disease

The basis for reversal of atherosclerosis is the initiation of a healing process in the artery wall that has been weakened by chronic vitamin deficiency. Optimum intake of Vitamin C and other ingredients is essential for the following reasons:

1   **Stability of the artery wall** through optimum collagen production. The collagen molecules in our body are proteins composed of amino acids. Collagen molecules differ from all other proteins in the body because they make particular use of the amino acids lysine and proline. An optimum supply of lysine, proline, and vitamin C is a decisive factor for the optimum regeneration of the connective tissue in the artery walls and, therefore, for a natural healing of cardiovascular disease.

2   **"Teflon" protection of the artery wall and reversal of fatty deposits in the artery walls.** Lipoproteins are the transport molecules by which cholesterol and other fat molecules circulate in the blood and are deposited in the artery walls. The primary therapeutic aim is to prevent fatty deposits in the artery wall and therefore to neutralize the stickiness of the lipoprotein molecules as well as to prevent their attachment to the inside of the artery walls. This can be achieved by means of "Teflon" substances for the artery walls. The natural amino acids lysine and proline form a protective "Teflon" layer around the lipoprotein(a) molecules. This prevents the deposition of more fat molecules in the artery wall and also releases lipoprotein molecules that had already been deposited there. Releasing fat molecules from the atherosclerotic deposits leads to a natural reversal of cardiovascular disease. These fat molecules are released in a natural way from the atherosclerotic plaques and transported to the liver. It is important to understand that this is a natural process, and complications that frequently accompany angioplasty and other mechanical procedures do not occur.

For this therapeutic approach we received the world's first patents for the natural prevention and reversal of cardiovascular diseases (see picture below).

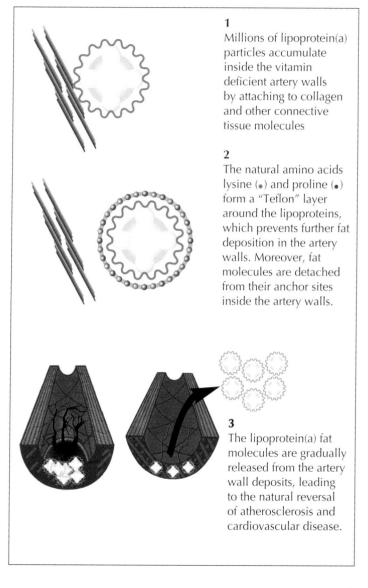

1
Millions of lipoprotein(a) particles accumulate inside the vitamin deficient artery walls by attaching to collagen and other connective tissue molecules

2
The natural amino acids lysine (•) and proline (•) form a "Teflon" layer around the lipoproteins, which prevents further fat deposition in the artery walls. Moreover, fat molecules are detached from their anchor sites inside the artery walls.

3
The lipoprotein(a) fat molecules are gradually released from the artery wall deposits, leading to the natural reversal of atherosclerosis and cardiovascular disease.

51

3 **Decrease of the "muscle cell tumor" in the artery wall.**
With an optimum supply of essential nutrients, the muscle
cells of the artery walls produce sufficient amounts of collagen, thereby guaranteeing optimum stability of the wall. In
contrast, vitamin deficiency leads to the production of
faulty collagen molecules by the arterial muscle cells.
Moreover, these muscle cells multiply themselves, forming
the atherosclerotic "tumor." My colleague, Dr. Aleksandra
Niedzwiecki and her colleagues investigated this mechanism in detail. They found that vitamin C, in particular, can
inhibit the growth of the atherosclerotic "tumor." In the
meantime, other studies have shown that vitamin E also has
this effect.

4 **Antioxidant protection in the bloodstream and artery
walls.** An additional mechanism accelerating the development of atherosclerosis, heart attacks and strokes, is biological oxidation. Free radicals, (aggressive molecules occur-
ring in cigarette smoke, car exhaust, and smog,) damage
the lipoproteins in the bloodstream and also the tissue of
the artery walls. This damage further extends the size of
atherosclerotic plaques. Vitamin C, vitamin E, beta
carotene, and other nutrients are among the strongest
natural antioxidants protecting the cardiovascular system
from oxidative damage.

High Cholesterol Levels and Other Secondary Risk Factors for Cardiovascular Disease

3

Cholesterol Is Only A Secondary Risk Factor

How Vitamins Can Help in Normalizing Cholesterol Levels

Clinical Studies With Vitamins Document the Natural Lowering of Risk Factors In Blood

Cholesterol Is Only A Secondary Risk Factor

Worldwide, hundreds of millions of people have elevated blood levels of cholesterol, triglycerides, LDL (low density lipoproteins), lipoprotein(a) and other risk factors. Contrary to what the pharmaceutical companies selling cholesterol-lowering drugs want to make you believe – there is nothing wrong with cholesterol levels of 220 or 240. At best cholesterol is a secondary risk factor because the primary risk factor determining your cardiovascular status is the weakness and instability of your blood vessel walls. Elevated blood levels of cholesterol and other blood risk factors are not the cause of cardiovascular diseases but are the consequence of developing disease.

Conventional medicine is limited to treating the symptoms of secondary risk factors. Drugs blocking the synthesis of cholesterol and other lipid-lowering agents are now being prescribed to millions of people These drugs are known to cause cancer and have other severe side effects. You should avoid them whenever you can.

Again, the reasons for elevated cholesterol levels are only partially understood by conventional medicine. Inherited disorders (genetic risk) and a high fat diet (dietary risk) are the two main reasons given in the textbooks of medicine. The most important reason is completely missing: a chronic deficiency of vitamins and other essential nutrients.

Modern Cellular Health provides a new understanding about the factors causing high blood levels of cholesterol and other secondary risk factors, as well as their natural prevention. Cholesterol, triglycerides, low density lipoproteins (LDL), lipoprotein(a) and other metabolic products are ideal repair factors, and their blood levels increase in response to a weakening of the artery walls. A chronic weakness of the blood vessel walls increases the demand for production of these repair molecules in the liver. An increased production of cholesterol and other repair factors in the liver increases the

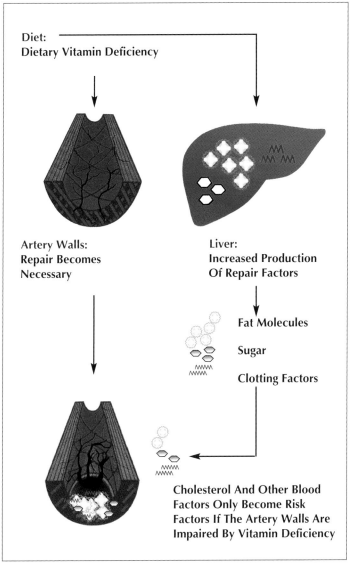

Diet:
Dietary Vitamin Deficiency

Artery Walls:
Repair Becomes
Necessary

Liver:
Increased Production
Of Repair Factors

Fat Molecules

Sugar

Clotting Factors

Cholesterol And Other Blood
Factors Only Become Risk
Factors If The Artery Walls Are
Impaired By Vitamin Deficiency

*ELEVATED CHOLESTEROL LEVELS ARE NOT THE CAUSE, BUT THE
CONSEQUENCE OF CARDIOVASCULAR DISEASE*

levels of these molecules in the bloodstream and over time renders them risk factors for cardiovascular disease. Thus, the primary measure for lowering cholesterol and other secondary risk factors in the bloodstream is to stabilize the artery walls and thereby lower the metabolic demand for increased production of these risk factors inside the body itself.

Therefore, it is not surprising that vitamins and other nutrients help in stabilizing the artery walls, and also, in parallel, help to decrease blood levels of cholesterol and other risk factors naturally.

My recommendations for people concerned with elevated cholesterol and other secondary risk factors. Lowering cholesterol without first stabilizing the artery walls is an insufficient and ill-fated cardiovascular therapy. Start as early as possible to increase the stability of your artery walls with essential nutrients to normalize blood levels of cholesterol and other isk factors.

What You Should Do:

1   Be aware that cholesterol is not the primary cause of heart disease. Be concerned with side-effects of cholesterol-lowering medication.

2   Help stabilize your artery walls and support the healing process with vitamins and other essential nutrients.

3   Eat more cereals, vegetables and other fiber-rich nutrition to "flush out" abundant cholesterol from your body naturally.

How Vitamins Can Help Patients With Elevated Cholesterol Levels

The blood levels of cholesterol respond quickly in most people who start nutritional supplementation. We already know the reason for this effect: this essential nutrient program helps in reducing the production of cholesterol and other secondary risk factors in the liver and thereby must lead to lower blood levels of these risk factors.

Interestingly, some people report an intermittent rise of cholesterol levels when they start taking vitamins. Because the rise of blood cholesterol levels is not the result of an increased cholesterol production, it has to come from other sources, primarily the atherosclerotic deposits in the artery walls. This important mechanism was first described by Dr. Constance Spittle in the medical journal The Lancet in 1972. She reported that vitamin supplementation in patients with existing cardiovascular disease frequently leads to a temporary increase of cholesterol levels in the blood. In contrast, the cholesterol levels of healthy test persons did not rise with vitamin supplementation.

The temporary rise of cholesterol is an additional sign of the healing process of the artery walls and the decrease of the fatty deposits. The mechanism described here is, of course, not only valid for cholesterol but also for triglycerides, LDL, lipoprotein(a), and other secondary risk factors which have accumulated over decades inside the artery walls and are now slowly released into the bloodstream.

My advice: Should your cholesterol levels rise when you start taking vitamins, it signifies the reversal of existing deposits. You should continue taking vitamins until, after several months, the blood level of cholesterol decreases below the initial values. A diet high in soluble fiber (e.g. in oat bran and other cereals) can further decrease cholesterol and other secondary risk factors in the blood.

Clinical Studies With Vitamins Document Natural Lowering of Risk Factors In Blood

We carried out clinical studies with a program of vitamins and other nutrients. The results of these pilot studies document the effectiveness and the safety of this natural health approach.

In one pilot study, fourteen patients with high cholesterol levels and other fat disorders followed the vitamin program for three months. During this period, their cholesterol levels decreased from an average of 293 mg/dl to 251 mg/dl accompanied by a decrease in triglyceride levels of 22%.

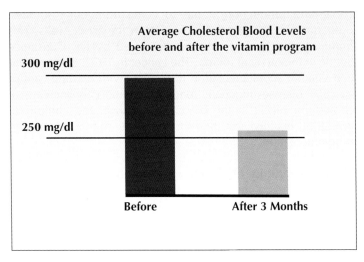

NATURAL CHOLESTEROL-LOWERING WITH VITAMIN PROGRAM

Most importantly, the average lipoprotein(a) levels decreased from 71 mg/dl to 62 mg/dl with use of vitamins. This fact is even more important, since there are currently no prescription drugs that are known to lower high lipoprotein(a) levels.

Moreover, no side-effects were reported with this natural health approach.

Clinical Studies With Critical Nutrients Document their Blood Risk Factors Lowering Effect

The effect of vitamin C on the blood levels of cholesterol has been documented in numerous clinical studies. More than 40 of these studies were evaluated by Dr. Hemilä from the University of Helsinki, Finland. In patients with high initial cholesterol values, (above 270 mg per deciliter) vitamin C supplementation decreased cholesterol levels up to 20%. In contrast, patients with low and medium initial values of cholesterol show only a slight cholesterollowering effect, or the levels stay the same.

Dr. Jacques and his colleagues showed that people taking at least 300 mg of Vitamin C per day had much higher HDL blood levels than people taking less than 120 mg per day. This is important since HDL (high-density lipoproteins) are fat-transporting molecules that pick up cholesterol and other fats from the artery walls and carry them back to the liver for removal. Dr. Hermann and his colleagues reported that vitamin E supplementation also increases HDL blood levels.

Further clinical studies show that other nutrients work synergistically with vitamin C to lower cholesterol and other blood fats. These components include vitamin B3 (nicotinic acid), vitamin B5 (pantothenate), vitamin E, carnitine, and other essential nutrients. (This synergistic effect is an important advantage compared to megadose intake of individual vitamins).

Clinical Study with	Reference
Vitamin C	Ginter, Harwood, Hemilä
Vitamin B-3	Altschul, Carlson, Guraker
Vitamin B-5	Avogaro, Cherchi, Gaddi
Vitamin E	Beamish, Hermann
Carnitine	Opie

Lipoprotein(a) – A Secondary Risk Factor – Ten Times More Dangerous Than Cholesterol

On the following pages I would like to describe in more detail lipoprotein(a), a secondary risk factor that is very important. The main function of lipoprotein(a) fulfills a variety of repair functions; for example during wound healing. However, if the artery wall is destabilized by a long- term vitamin deficiency, lipoprotein(a) turns into a risk factor ten times more dangerous than cholesterol. Let's have a closer look at how lipoprotein(a) molecules differ from other fat molecules.

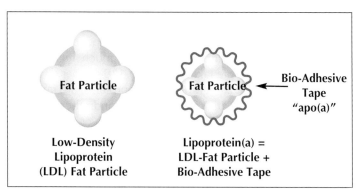

COMPARISON BETWEEN LDL AND LIPOPROTEIN(A)

Cholesterol and triglycerides do not swim in the blood like fat swims in soup. Thousands of cholesterol molecules are packed together with other fat molecules in tiny round globules called lipoproteins. Millions of these fat-transporting vehicles circulate in our body at any given time. The best known among these lipoproteins are high-density lipoproteins (HDL, or "good cholesterol") and low-density lipoproteins (LDL, or "bad cholesterol").

LDL-Cholesterol. Most cholesterol molecules in the blood are transported in millions of LDL particles. By carrying cholesterol and other fat molecules to our body cells, LDL is a very useful vehicle for supplying nutrients to these cells. LDL has been named the "bad cholesterol" because, researchers believed that LDL was primarily responsible for the fatty deposits in the artery walls. (This theory is now out of date).

Lipoprotein(a) is an LDL particle with an additional adhesive protein surrounding it. This biological adhesive tape is named apoprotein(a), or abreviated, apo(a). The letter (a) could in fact stand for "adhesive." The adhesive apo(a) makes the lipoprotein(a) fat globule one of the stickiest particles in our body. Together with my colleagues at Hamburg University, I conducted the most comprehensive studies on lipoprotein(a) in the artery wall. These studies showed that the atherosclerotic lesions in human arteries are largely composed of lipoprotein(a) rather than LDL molecules. Moreover, the size of the atherosclerotic lesions paralleled the amount of lipoprotein(a) particles deposited in the arteries. These findings have been confirmed in a series of further clinical studies.

Lipoprotein(a) blood levels vary greatly between one individual and another. What do we know about the factors influencing the lipoprotein(a) levels in your blood? Lipoprotein(a) levels are primarily determined by inheritance. Special diets do not influence lipoprotein(a) blood levels. Moreover, none of the presently available lipid-lowering prescription drugs lower lipoprotein(a) blood concentrations. The only substances that have thus far been shown to lower lipoprotein(a) levels are vitamins. Professor L.A. Carlson showed that two to four grams of vitamin B3 (nicotinic acid) per day could lower lipoprotein(a) levels up to 36%. Because high levels of nicotinic acid can cause skin rash, you are well advised to increase daily intake of nicotinic acid slowly.

Our own research showed that vitamin C alone, or in combination with lower dosages of nicotinic acid, may also reduce the production of lipoproteins and thereby on decreasing lipoprotein blood levels. Together with the "Teflon" agents lysine and proline, vitamin C and nicotinic acid can considerably reduce the cardiovascular risk associated with lipoprotein(a) levels.

What Does Medicine Today Know About Lipoprotein(a)?

- Lipoprotein(a), not LDL, is the most important fat particle responsible for the deposition of cholesterol and other fats in the artery walls.
- Because of its sticky properties, lipoprotein(a) is one of the most effective repair molecules in the artery wall and, with ongoing vitamin deficiency, becomes one of the most dangerous risk factors for atherosclerosis and cardiovascular disease.
- A reevaluation of the Framingham Heart Study, the largest cardiovascular risk factor study ever conducted, showed that lipoprotein(a) is a ten-fold greater risk factor for heart disease than cholesterol or LDL-cholesterol.

Lipoprotein(a) is a particularly interesting molecule because of its inverse relationship to vitamin C. The following discovery triggered my interest in vitamin research: lipoprotein(a) molecules are primarily found in humans and a few animal species unable to produce vitamin C. In contrast, animals able to produce optimum amounts of vitamin C do not need lipoprotein(a) Lipoprotein(a) molecules apparently compensate for many properties of vitamin C such as wound healing and blood vessel repair. In 1990, I published the details of this important discovery in the Proceedings of the National Academy of Sciences and invited Linus Pauling as co-author for this publication.

The Cholesterol – Heart Disease Myth

The leading medical speculation about the origin of cardiovascular disease is as follows: high levels of cholesterol and risk factors circulating in the blood would damage the blood vessel walls and lead to atherosclerotic deposits. According to this hypothesis, lowering of cholesterol is the primary measure to prevent cardiovascular disease. The driving force behind this theory is the the multi-billion dollar market of cholesterol-lowering drugs. The following facts are little known:

In the 1970's, the World Health Organization (WHO) conducted an international study to answer the question of whether cholesterol-lowering drugs can decrease the risk of heart attacks. Thousands of the participants received the cholesterol-lowering drug Clofibrate. This study could not be completed because those who took the cholesterol-lowering drug experienced too many side effects.

In the early 1980's, a large-scale study of more than 3,800 American men made headline news. This study tested whether the cholesterol-lowering drug Cholestyramine can lower the risk of heart attacks. One study group took up to 24 grams (24,000 milligrams) of Cholestyramine every day over several years. The control group of this study took the same amount of placebos (ineffective control substance). The result of this study was that in the cholesterol-lowering drug group the same number of people died as in the control group. Accidents and suicides were very frequent among patients taking this cholesterol-lowering drug. Irrespective of these facts, those interested in marketing the drug decided to promote this study as a success. The fact that there were fewer incidences of heart attacks in the drug group was marketed as a confirmation of the cholesterol-heart attack-hypothesis. Hardly anyone bothered with the actual death figures of this study. In the late 1980's, a new group of cholesterol-lowering drugs was introduced, the "statins". Later it was determined that these drugs not only lower the production of cholesterol, but also the production of carriers of cellular energy (Coenzyme Q-10). Professor Karl Folkers, from the University of Texas in Austin, rang alarm bells in the *Proceedings of the National Academy of Science*. He reported that patients with existing heart failure taking these new cholesterol-lowering drugs could experience muscle pain, liver damage and life-threatening deterioration of their heart functions.

A giant blow for the cholesterol-lowering drug industry came on January 6, 1996. On that day the *Journal of the American Medical Association* published an article entitled "Carcinogenicity of Cholesterol-lowering Drugs." Dr. T.B. Newman and Dr. S.B. Hulley from San Francisco University Medical School showed that most of the cholesterol-lowering drugs on the market, namely statins and fibrates, cause cancer in test animals taking levels equal to humans. The authors raised the legitimate question: "How could it be that the U.S. Food and Drug Administration, (FDA), allowed these drugs to be sold to millions of people?" The answer is: "The pharmaceutical companies manufacturing these drugs downplayed the importance of these side effects and thereby removed any obstacles for approval."

Since the first publication of this book, millions of people have learned that animals don't get heart attacks because they produce vitamin C - not because they have low cholesterol levels. Heart attacks are the primary result of vitamin deficiencies - not of elevated cholesterol. It is clear that cholesterol-lowering drugs and many other drugs will eventually be replaced by essential nutrients The time needed will depend on one factor only: How fast information about the connection between scurvy and cardiovascular disease can spread.

Important Nutrients to Maintain Optimum Cholesterol and Fat Metabolism

The following cellular bioenergy factors are important to optimize cell metabolism and maintain healthy cholesterol levels in the blood:

- **Vitamin C:** protection and natural healing of the artery walls, lowering increased production of cholesterol and other secondary risk factors in the liver and elevated blood levels of these secondary risk factors.

- **Vitamin E:** anti-oxidant protection for blood fats and millions of body cells.

- **Vitamin B1:** optimizing cellular metabolism, particularly delivery of bioenergy.

- **Vitamin B2:** optimizing cellular metabolism, particularly delivery of bioenergy.

- **Vitamin B3:** lowering elevated production of cholesterol and lipoproteins in the liver.

- **Vitamin B5:** structural component of the central metabolic molecule of cells (coenzyme A), optimized metabolic burning of fat molecules.

- **Vitamin B6, biotin and folic acid:** counteracting increased levels of the risk factor homocysteine, optimizing metabolism of cells.

- **Carnitine:** optimizing cellular metabolism of fats, lowering of triglyceride levels.

Why Bears Are Not Extinct

If anyone among my readers still thinks that cholesterol may cause heart attacks, I would like to share the following facts: Bears and millions of other hibernating animals have average cholesterol levels of over 400 milligrams per deciliter. Indeed, if cholesterol were the culprit causing heart attacks and strokes, bears and millions of other hibernating animals would have long been extinct. The reason that bears are still among us is simple: they produce high amounts of vitamin C in their bodies, stabilize their artery walls.

The fact that bears are not extinct proves:

1   Elevated cholesterol blood levels are not the primary cause of atherosclerosis, heart attacks and strokes.
2   Achieving and maintaining stability of the artery walls through optimum vitamin supply is more important than lowering cholesterol and other risk factors in the blood stream.
3   Cholesterol and other repair factors in the blood stream can only become risk factors if the artery walls are weakened by chronic vitamin deficiency.

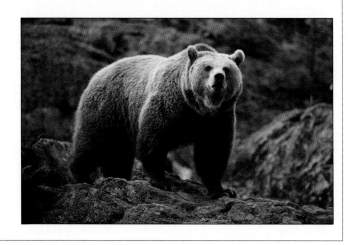

4

High Blood
Pressure

The Facts About High Blood Pressure

How Vitamins Help In Optimizing Blood Pressure

Scientific Information About Blood Pressure
And Vitamins

Further Clinical Studies With Vitamins And
Blood Pressure

The Facts About High Blood Pressure

Worldwide several hundred million people suffer from high blood pressure conditions. The spread of this disease is largely due to the fact that, until now, the causes for high blood pressure have been insufficiently understood.

Conventional medicine concedes that the causes of high blood pressure are unknown in over 90% of patients. The frequent medical diagnosis, "essential hypertension" was established to describe the high blood pressure conditions in which the causes remain unknown. Accordingly, conventional medicine is confined to treating the symptoms of this disease. Beta-blockers, diuretics and other high blood pressure medications target the symptoms of high blood pressure, but not its underlying cause.

Modern Cellular Health provides a breakthrough in our understanding of the causes, prevention and adjunct therapy of high blood pressure conditions. The main cause of high blood pressure is a chronic deficiency of essential nutrients in millions of artery wall cells. Among other functions, these cells are responsible for the production of "relaxing factors" which decrease vascular wall tension and keep the blood pressure in a normal range. The natural amino acid arginine, vitamin C and other nutrients contribute to optimum availability of these artery wall relaxing factors. In contrast, chronic deficiency of these essential nutrients can result in spasms and thickening of the blood vessel walls, and can eventually elevate blood pressure.

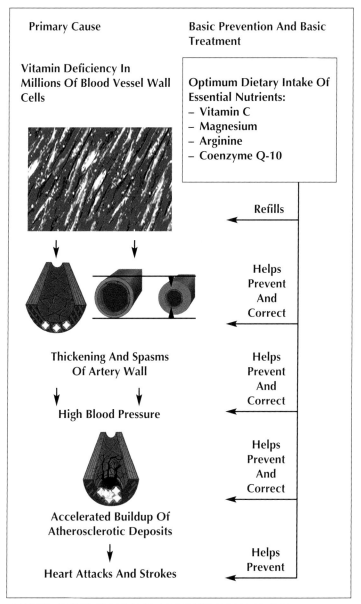

*CAUSES, PREVENTION AND ADJUNCT TREATMENT IN
NORMALIZING BLOOD PRESSURE*

73

How Vitamins Help in Optimizing Blood Pressure

Thousands of people benefit from learning about the benefits of nutrients in normalizing blood pressure Following are two typical letters.

Dear Dr. Rath,
About 8 weeks ago I was introduced to a fiber product for the reduction of my cholesterol, which had reached 260 in spite of efforts to get it down. After being on that product about 2 and a half weeks, I realized that my blood pressure was going up. **I have been on blood pressure medication for essential hypertension since my teen years.** I supposed that it was due to the energy I was feeling from the fiber formula.

Then I heard vitamins and nutrients can help in lowering blood pressure. I immediately started on this program. **Within two weeks my blood pressure had gone from 145/150 over 90/96 to 130/82 - sometimes a bit higher if I am really busy!** I noticed a lessening of a feeling of chest pressure also, and I could breathe deeper.

Sincerely,   S.S.

Dear Dr. Rath,

I have been following the cardiovascular vitamin program for five months. In the meantime my doctor reduced my blood pressure medication by half so I can honestly say I'm now taking half the medication than five months ago. I am maintaining blood pressure average of 120/78. Thrilled? You'd better believe it! Next goal: no medication at all. Thank you again.

Sincerely,   L.M.

Scientific Information About Blood Pressure and Vitamins

We carried out clinical studies with Dr. Rath's Vitamin Program in patients with high blood pressure. The results of these studies document the effectiveness and safety of this natural health approach.

In a pilot study ten patients with high blood pressure followed the vitamin program for four months. After eight weeks their average blood pressure decreased from 185 over 105 to 144 over 81. Thus, both blood pressure values (systolic and diastolic) decreased more than 20%. The blood pressure in these patients was almost normalized naturally during this study.

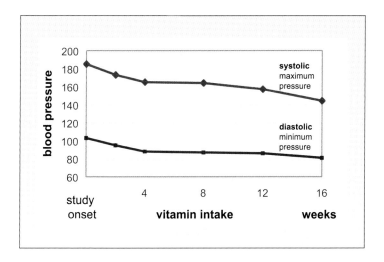

The results of this and other natural health studies are even more important because most prescription blood pressure medications affect only the <u>symptoms</u> of the disease. The natural ingredients in the vitamin program help to relax the blood vessel walls and thereby help normalize blood pressure by addressing the root of the problem.

75

Further Clinical Studies With Vitamins And Blood Pressure

Various clinical studies show that different nutrients are important for normalizing blood pressure conditions. The following table summarizes some of the most significant studies:

Nutrients	Blood Pressure-Lowering	Reference
Vitamin C	5% to 10%	McCarron
Coenzyme Q-10	10% to 15%	Digiesi
Magnesium	10% to 15%	Turlapaty, Widman
Arginine	more than 10%	Korbut

It is important to note that in all these studies the natural components helped to normalize the blood pressure but did not cause a too-low blood pressure situation. This is another advantage compared to conventional medication, where over-dosing frequently leads to decreased blood circulation, dizziness, and other health problems.

Important Nutrients in Normalizing Blood Pressure

The following bioenergy cell factors are important for optimal cell metabolism and normalizing blood pressure:

- **Vitamin C:** decreased tension of the artery wall, increased supply of relaxing factors, lowering of elevated blood pressure.

- **Vitamin E:** anti-oxidant protection, protection of cell membranes and blood components.

- **Arginine:** improved production of "relaxing factors", decreased tension of the artery walls, lowering of elevated blood pressure.

- **Magnesium:** optimizing cellular metabolism of minerals, decreased tension of the blood vessel walls, lowering of high blood pressure.

- **Calcium:** optimizing mineral metabolism, decreased tension of the artery walls, lowering of high blood pressure.

- **Bioflavonoids:** catalysts which, among others, improve the efficacy of vitamin C.

Notes

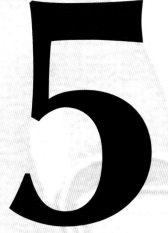

Heart Failure

5

The Facts About Heart Failure

Vitamins in Optimizing Heart Muscle Function

Clinical Evidence that Vitamins and Other Nutrients Can Optimize Heart Muscle Function

Further Clinical Studies with Vitamins

Problems with Incomplete Treatment of Heart Failure

The Facts About Heart Failure

Tens of millions of people worldwide are currently suffering from heart failure, resulting in shortness of breath, edema, and fatigue. The number of heart failure patients has tripled over the last four decades. The epidemic spread of this disease is largely due to the fact that until now the causes of heart failure have been insufficiently understood, if at all. In some cases heart failure is the result of a heart attack; in most cases, however, such as cardiomyopathies, heart failure develops without any prior cardiac event.

Conventional medicine is largely confined to treating the symptoms of heart failure. Diuretic drugs flush out the water that is retained in the body because of the weak pumping function of the heart. Still, insufficient understanding of the causes of heart failure also explains the unfavorable prognosis of this disease. Five years after a heart failure condition is diagnosed, only 50% of the patients are alive. For many patients with heart failure, a heart transplant operation is the last resort. Most heart failure patients, however, die without ever having the option of such an operation.

Cellular Health provides a breakthrough in understanding of the causes, prevention, and adjunct treatment of heart failure. The primary cause of heart failure is a deficiency of vitamins and other essential nutrients that provide bioenergy to millions of heart muscle cells. These muscle cells are responsible for the contraction of the heart muscle and for optimum pumping of blood for circulation. Deficiencies of vitamins and other essential nutrients impair the pumping performance of the heart, resulting in shortness of breath, edema, and fatigue.

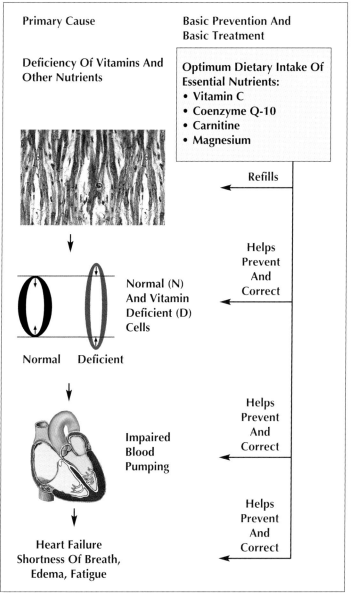

Primary Cause

Basic Prevention And
Basic Treatment

Deficiency Of Vitamins And
Other Nutrients

Optimum Dietary Intake Of
Essential Nutrients:
• Vitamin C
• Coenzyme Q-10
• Carnitine
• Magnesium

Refills

Normal (N)
And Vitamin
Deficient (D)
Cells

Normal   Deficient

Helps
Prevent
And
Correct

Impaired
Blood
Pumping

Helps
Prevent
And
Correct

Heart Failure
Shortness Of Breath,
Edema, Fatigue

Helps
Prevent
And
Correct

CAUSES, PREVENTION AND TREATMENT OF HEART FAILURE

81

Vitamins in Optimizing Heart Muscle Function

Vitamins and other nutrients are important for optimum function of the heart muscle. Following are two examples of patient letters:

Heart Transplant Operation Cancelled

Dear Dr. Rath,

Our sister-in-law was diagnosed with **congestive heart failure** and was told by her physician to go home and get her affairs in order, sell her home and prepare to move into a nursing home because she was only going to get worse and wouldn't be able to care for herself. **Her chest was full of fluids, she had to sleep sitting up, she was too weak to walk and her legs were swelling.**

She started using nutritional supplements late in February, and **in three weeks she was feeling well enough to go out for dinner, get her hair done and put her house on the market.** She has since moved into a nice retirement home and she goes everywhere the bus goes. She is so grateful, she has been given her life back and never wants to be without your vitamin program.

Sincerely, R.A

After visiting with a heart failure patient and his cardiologist, I personally wrote the following report about the health improvement of this patient. From now on, heart failure patients around the world can benefit from vitamin intake which provides essential bioenergy to their heart muscle cells.

G.P. is an entrepreneur in his fifties. **Three years ago his life was changed by a sudden occurrence of heart failure,** a weakness of the heart muscle leading to a decreased pumping function and to an enlargement of the heart chambers. The patient could no longer fully meet his professional obligations and had to give up all his sports activities. **On some days he felt so weak that he couldn't climb stairs and he had to hold his drinking glass with both hands.** Because of the continued weak pumping function of the heart and the unfavorable prognosis of this disease, his cardiologist recommended a heart transplant operation: "I recommend you get a new heart."

At this point the patient started to take nutritional supplements. His physical strength improved gradually. **Soon he could again fulfill his professional obligations on a regular basis and was able to enjoy daily bicycle rides. Two months after starting to follow my recommendations his cardiologist noted a decrease in size of the previously enlarged heart in the echocardiography examination, another sign of a recovering heart muscle.** One month later the patient was able to take a business trip abroad and he could attend to his business affairs without any physical limitations.

Clinical Evidence that Vitamins and Other Nutrients can Optimize Heart Muscle Function

A clinical study with a vitamin program documented improvement in the heart pumping function in patients with heart failure. This clinical pilot study included six patients aged 40 to 66. The heart performance of these patients was first measured by **echocardiography (ultrasound examination of the heart)**. This test measures how much blood the heart pumps into the circulation with every heartbeat (ejection fraction). In addition, the physical performance of the patients was assessed with a treadmill ergometer.

Then the patients followed a vitamin program in addition to their regular medication. After two months on this program, echocardiographic and ergometric control examinations were conducted. With this nutritional supplement program, the ejection fraction and the physical performance increased on average by 20%. Thus, supplementation with vitamins was able to improve heart performance beyond any prescription drug tested thus far.

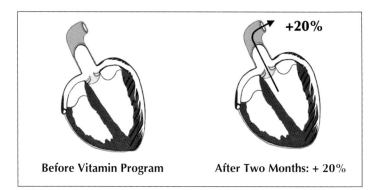

| Before Vitamin Program | After Two Months: + 20% |

VITAMIN PROGRAM IMPROVES HEART PUMPING BY 20%

In another clinical pilot study, ten patients with heart failure followed the vitamin program for six months. The severity of the heart failure condition was determined using the New York Heart Association (NYHA)scale. 1 = slight physical impairment, normal life possible; 2 = ability to work is moderately impaired; 3 = ability to work is severely impaired (generally: disability); 4 = severely ill.

At the beginning of the study, seven out of ten patients suffered from severe physical impairment and three from moderate impairment. After six months of taking vitamins, 50% of the patients could lead a normal life again. They no longer suffered from shortness of breath and other symptoms of heart failure in their daily work. Patients two and three admitted that they did not follow the vitamin program. They did not show any improvement of their condition.

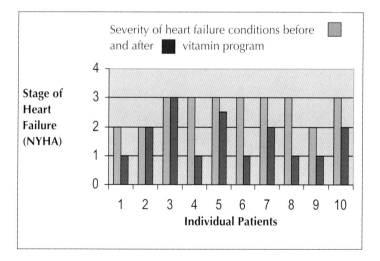

Vitamins and other nutrients function as bioenergy carriers to millions of heart muscle cells. Thus, during this study the most common symptoms of heart failure improved in those patients taking vitamins:

- Water retention (leg swelling) completely disappeared.
- Shortness of breath decreased more than 70%.
- Frequent urination decreased by 40%.
- Severe fatigue disappeared entirely.
- Rapid heart beat also disappeared completely.

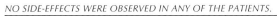

NO SIDE-EFFECTS WERE OBSERVED IN ANY OF THE PATIENTS.

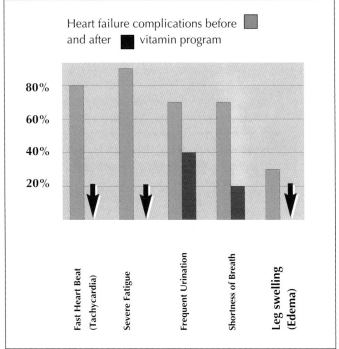

The results of these pilot studies document the effectiveness and the safety of this natural health approach.

Further Clinical Studies With Vitamins

Numerous clinical studies have demonstrated the value of vitamins and other nutrients in such conditions as shortness of breath, edema, and other heart failure symptoms.

The most comprehensive clinical studies tested Coenzyme Q-10 and carnitine, carrier molecules of bioenergy in millions of heart muscle cells. For example, Professors Langsjoen, Folkers, and their colleagues from the University of Texas in Austin showed that heart failure patients taking Coenzyme Q-10 in addition to their regular medication could significantly improve their survival chances.

After three years, 75% of those patients who took Coenzyme Q-10 in addition to their regular medication were still alive, whereas of those patients who took only their regular medication, 25% were still alive. Statistically, every second patient in this study owed his or her life to Coenzyme Q-10 supplementation.

Besides Coenzyme Q-10 and Carnitine, other important natural substances optimize the metabolism of heart muscle cells. This also explains the impressive success of our clinical pilot study in heart failure patients who started on a program comprised of vitamins, minerals and other nutrients. The following table summarizes the most important clinical studies with coenzyme Q10 and Carnitine.

Nutrient	Reference
Coenzyme Q-10	Folkers, Langsjoen
Carnitine	Ghidini

Problems with Incomplete Treatment of Heart Failure

For decades, bias and skepticism have prevented medicine from identifying the primary cause of heart failure. Today, we know that a deficiency of vitamins and other essential nutrients in millions of heart muscle cells is the primary cause of heart failure. The conventional treatment of heart failure patients is an example of how an incomplete understanding of the causes of a disease at the level of cells can lead to a vicious cycle in which therapeutic measures can contribute to aggravating the health problem.

A chronic deficiency of nutrients in heart muscle cells causes decreased pumping function. This frequently leads to lower blood pressure and an impaired blood supply to different organs in the body, e.g., the kidneys. The primary role of the kidneys is to filter excess water from the blood. With impaired blood flow through the kidneys, less water is filtered and instead of leaving the body via urine, fluid accumulates in the tissue of legs, lungs and other parts of the body (edema). In order to eliminate the abundant body water, doctors prescribe diuretic medication.

At this point a vicious cycle is triggered in the conventional therapy of heart failure. Diuretics not only increase water elimination from the body but also wash out water soluble vitamins, such as vitamin C and B vitamins, as well as important minerals and trace elements. Since vitamin deficiency is already the main cause of heart failure, diuretic medication further aggravates the underlying cause. This is why heart failure patients have such a short life expectancy.

The treatment of heart failure patients with diuretics alone is incomplete. Supplementation with essential nutrients is critical. If you are a patient suffering from heart failure, you should talk with your doctor about it.

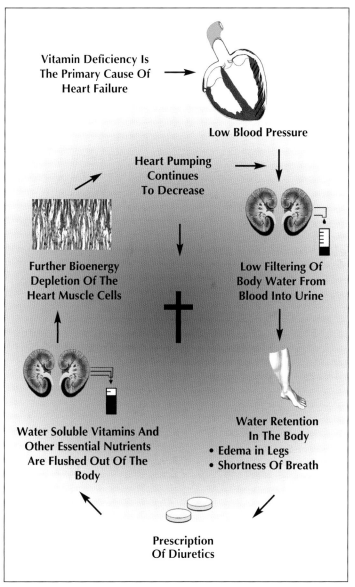

Vitamin Deficiency Is
The Primary Cause Of
Heart Failure

Low Blood Pressure

Heart Pumping
Continues
To Decrease

Further Bioenergy
Depletion Of The
Heart Muscle Cells

Low Filtering Of
Body Water From
Blood Into Urine

Water Retention
In The Body
• Edema in Legs
• Shortness Of Breath

Water Soluble Vitamins And
Other Essential Nutrients
Are Flushed Out Of The
Body

Prescription
Of Diuretics

*THE VICIOUS CYCLE RESULTING FROM THE INCOMPLETE
TREATMENT OF HEART FAILURE*

Nutrients Important for Optimum Heart Muscle Function

The following cellular bioenergy factors are important for optimum function of heart muscle cells and the heart muscle.

- **Vitamin C:** energy supply for the metabolism of each cell, supplies the bioenergy carrier molecules of the Vitamin B group with life-saving bioenergy.

- **Vitamin E:** anti-oxidative protection, protection of the cell membranes.

- **Vitamin B1, B2, B3, B5, B6, B12 and biotin:** bioenergy carriers of cellular metabolism, particularly for the heart muscle cells, improved heart function and heart pumping, improved physical endurance.

- **Coenzyme Q10:** most important element of the "respiration chain" of each cell, plays a particular role for improved heart muscle function because of the high bioenergy demand in the heart muscle cells.

- **Carnitine:** improved supply of bioenergy for the "power plants" (mitochondria) of millions of cells.

- **Taurine:** Taurine is a natural amino acid, its lack in the heart muscle cells is a particular frequent cause of heart failure.

My advice for patients with heart failure: Inform your doctor about the importance of these nutrients for your heart conditions. You can take these essential nutrients in addition to your regular medication. Do not stop or alter your regular medication on your own.

6

Irregular Heartbeat (Arrhythmia)

Facts About Irregular Heartbeat

Vitamins in Optimizing Heart Pumping Function

Clinical Studies In Arrhythmia

Facts About Irregular Heartbeat

Over 100 million people worldwide suffer from an irregular heartbeat. Irregular heartbeat is caused by a disturbance in the creation or conduction of the electrical impulse responsible for a heartbeat. In some cases, these disturbances are caused by a damaged area of the heart muscle, e.g., after a heart attack. The textbooks of medicine, however, admit that the causes for most irregular heartbeat remain unknown. No wonder that irregular heartbeat conditions are spreading like an epidemic on a worldwide scale.

Conventional medicine has invented its own diagnostic terms to cover the fact that it does not know the origin of most arrhythmias. "Paroxysmal" arrhythmia means "causes unknown." As a direct consequence, the therapeutic options of conventional medicine are confined to treating the symptoms of irregular heartbeat. Beta-blockers, calcium antagonists, and other anti-arrhythmic drugs are given to patients in the hope that the incidents of irregular heartbeat decrease.

Arrhythmias with long pauses between heartbeats are dealt with by implanting a pacemaker. In other cases, heart muscle tissue that creates or conducts uncoordinated electrical impulses is cauterized (burned) and thereby eliminated. Lacking an understanding of the primary cause of irregular heartbeat, the therapeutic approaches by conventional medicine are not specific and therefore frequently fail.

Modern Cellular Health now provides a decisive breakthrough in our understanding of the causes, prevention, and adjunct therapy of irregular heartbeat. The most frequent cause of irregular heartbeat is a chronic deficiency in vitamins and other essential nutrients in millions of electrical heart muscle cells. Long term, these deficiencies of essential nutrients directly cause, or aggravate, disturbances in the creation or conduction of the electrical impulses triggering the heartbeat. Thus, the primary method for preventing and correcting an

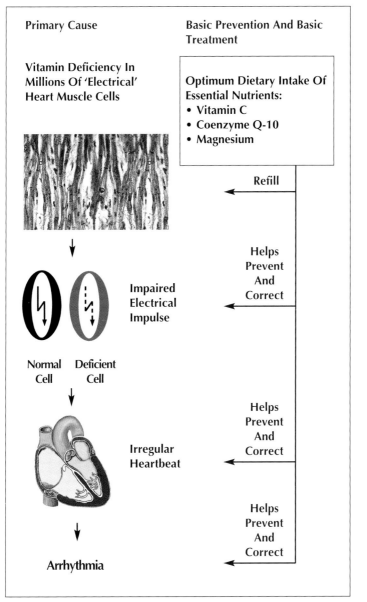

Primary Cause

Basic Prevention And Basic Treatment

Vitamin Deficiency In Millions Of 'Electrical' Heart Muscle Cells

Optimum Dietary Intake Of Essential Nutrients:
- **Vitamin C**
- **Coenzyme Q-10**
- **Magnesium**

Refill

Impaired Electrical Impulse

Helps Prevent And Correct

Normal Cell   Deficient Cell

Irregular Heartbeat

Helps Prevent And Correct

Arrhythmia

Helps Prevent And Correct

CAUSES, PREVENTION AND TREATMENT OF IRREGULAR HEARTBEAT

irregular heartbeat is an optimum supply of vitamins and other essential nutrients.

Vitamins in Optimizing Heart Pumping Function

Please share the following letters and this book with anyone you know suffering from irregular heartbeat. By doing so, you may be able to improve the quality of life of a person, or even save a life.

Dear Dr. Rath:

Two months ago I was experiencing loud heartbeats, tachycardia and irregular beating of the heart. I saw my doctor who promptly put me on an anti-arrhythmic drug. I can honestly say the medication did me absolutely no good.

Then, I started using vitamins. What a smart decision that was! **Within a few days, the tachycardia stopped and I've not experienced any loud or irregular heartbeats.** It's like a miracle. It must be the combination of nutrients because I had been taking Coenzyme Q10 separately from my regular vitamins. Because of your research, I'm able to continue working.

Sincerely, B.M.

Dear Dr. Rath:

In February I introduced my 74 year old grandmother to your book. **Her slow and irregular heart beat had led her doctor to begin preliminary preparations to install a pacemaker.**

After about three weeks of using vitamins her heart action was sufficiently improved to cause the doctor to postpone this procedure. This lady is now a faithful follower of natural health programs and, although she faces other medical challenges, her heart condition continues to improve, and the use of a pacemaker is no longer being considered.

Sincerely, K.C

Dear Dr. Rath:

I am 54 years of age and have had a very irregular heartbeat for at least 20 years. This was diagnosed as second degree electrical heart block. I have never taken any medication for this. I have had a stress test done approximately every 2 years and the heart block has shown up on the EKG. I was told that as long as my heartbeat became regular when I excercised that I did not need any other treatment.

In June I even went back to the doctor where I had my last EKG done so there would be a basis for comparison. **The doctor found that there was no longer any arrhythmia seen. I have enclosed a copy of his report.** I am sure that the vitamin program I have been taking is responsible for the correction of my irregular heartbeat, as I had not changed my lifestyle in any other respect

Sincerely, T.H

Clinical Studies in Arrhythmia

In addition to individual patient reports, clinical studies have documented the health benefits of various nutrients in patients with irregular heartbeat. The following table summarizes some of the most important clinical studies in this area:

Nutrient	References
Magnesium	England, Turlapaty
Carnitine	Rizzon

Irregular heartbeat and heart failure are both facilitated by a lack of bioenergy molecules in millions of heart muscle cells. Vitamins, minerals and specific bioenergy factors help millions of heart muscle cells to function properly.

My recommendations: Inform your doctor about the importance of these nutrients for your heart conditions.

Take these essential nutrients in addition to your regular medication. Do not stop or alter your regular medication on your own.

Any changes of anti-arrhythmic medication can have serious consequences for your heartbeat and should be done only in consultation with your doctor.

Important Nutrients for Optimum Heart Pumping Function

The following cellular bioenergy factors *in addition to* regular medication can help in optimizing pumping performance of the heart:

- **Vitamin C:** energy supply for the metabolism of each cell, supplies the bioenergy carrier molecules of the Vitamin B group with life-saving bio-energy.

- **Vitamin E:** anti-oxidative protection, protection of the cell membranes.

- **Vitamin B1, B2, B3, B5, B6, B12 and biotin:** bio-energy carriers of cellular metabolism, particularly for the heart muscle cells, improved heart function and heart pumping, improved physical endurance.

- **Coenzyme Q10:** most important element of the "respiration chain" of each cell, plays a particular role for improved heart muscle function because of the high bioenergy demand in the heart muscle cells.

- **Carnitine:** improved supply of bioenergy for the "power plants" (mitochondria) of millions of cells.

- **Taurine:** Taurine is a natural amino acid; its lack in the heart muscle cells is a frequent cause of heart failure.

My advice to patients with irregular heartbeat: Start as soon as possible with vitamin program and inform your doctor about it. Take these essential vitamins *in addition* to your regular medication. Do not stop or alter your regular medication on your own.

99

Diabetes

7

The Facts About Vitamins and Adult Diabetes

Cardiovascular Complications in Diabetes

Clinical Studies Document Effectiveness of Vitamins in Diabetic Conditions

The Facts About Adult Diabetes

Worldwide over one hundred million people are suffering from diabetes. Diabetic disorders have a genetic background and are divided into two types: juvenile and adult onset diabetes. Juvenile diabetes is generally caused by an inborn defect that leads to insufficient insulin in the body and requires regular insulin injections to control blood sugar levels. The majority of diabetic patients, however, develop this disease as adults. Adult forms of diabetes also have a genetic background. The causes, however, that trigger the outbreak of the disease in these patients at any stage of their adult lives, have been unknown. It is, therefore, not surprising that diabetes is yet another disease that is still expanding on a worldwide scale.

Conventional medicine is confined to treating the symptoms of adult diabetes by lowering elevated blood sugar levels. However, cardiovascular diseases and other diabetic complications occur even in those patients with controlled blood sugar levels. Thus, lowering of blood sugar levels is a necessary but an insufficient and incomplete treatment of diabetic disorders.

Modern Cellular Health now provides a breakthrough in our understanding of the causes, the prevention, and the adjunct therapy of adult diabetes. Adult onset diabetes is frequently caused or aggravated by a deficiency of certain vitamins and other essential nutrients in millions of cells in the pancreas, the liver, and the blood vessel walls.This deficiency of nutrients can trigger a diabetic metabolism and the onset of adult diabetes in people with a genetic predisposition to diabetic disorders. Vice versa, optimum intake of vitamins and other nutrients can help prevent the onset of adult diabetes and correct, at least in part, existing diabetes and its complications.

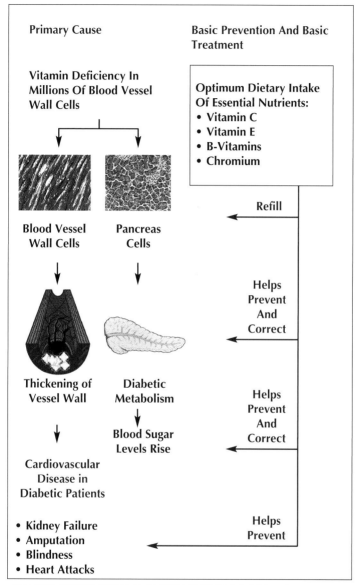

Primary Cause

Basic Prevention And Basic Treatment

Vitamin Deficiency In Millions Of Blood Vessel Wall Cells

Optimum Dietary Intake Of Essential Nutrients:
- **Vitamin C**
- **Vitamin E**
- **B-Vitamins**
- **Chromium**

Refill

Blood Vessel Wall Cells

Pancreas Cells

Helps Prevent And Correct

Thickening of Vessel Wall

Diabetic Metabolism

Blood Sugar Levels Rise

Helps Prevent And Correct

Cardiovascular Disease in Diabetic Patients

- Kidney Failure
- Amputation
- Blindness
- Heart Attacks

Helps Prevent

CAUSES, PREVENTION AND TREATMENT OF CARDIOVASCULAR COMPLICATIONS IN DIABETES

How Diabetic Cardiovascular Disease Develops

The key to understanding cardiovascular disease in diabetics is the similarity in the molecular structure of vitamin C and sugar (glucose) molecules. This similarity leads to a confusion at the level of cells with severe consequences:

Column A on the next page shows that the cells of our blood vessel walls contain tiny biological pumps specialized for pumping sugar and vitamin C molecules from the blood stream into the blood vessel wall. In a healthy person, these pumps transport an optimum amount of sugar and vitamin C molecules into the blood vessel wall, enabling normal function of the wall and preventing cardiovascular disease.

Column B shows the situation in a diabetic patient. Because of the high sugar concentration in the blood, the sugar+vitamin C pumps are overloaded with sugar molecules. This leads to an overload of sugar and, simultaneously, to a deficiency of vitamin C inside the blood vessel walls. The consequence of these mechanisms is a thickening of the walls throughout the blood vessel pipeline, putting any organ at risk for infarctions.

Column C shows the decisive measure for preventing cardiovascular complications in diabetes. An optimum daily intake of vitamins and other nutrients, in particular of vitamin C, helps to normalize the imbalance between vitamin and sugar metabolism.

Diabetes is an inherited condition, but the trigger for the onset of this disease is a chronic deficiency of vitamin C and other essential nutrients. Based on this new understanding, optimum vitamin supply will soon become the basic preventive and therapeutic measure for diabetes.

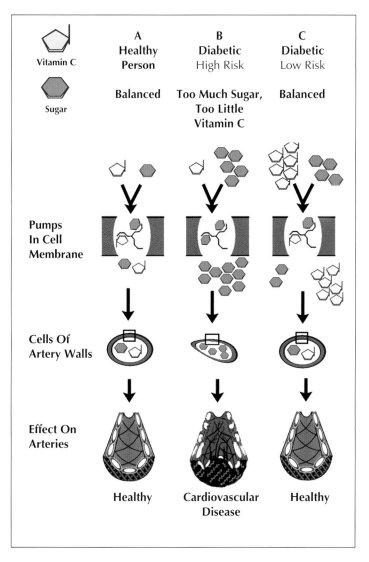

VITAMIN C IS THE BASIC NUTRIENT FOR DIABETIC PATIENTS IN PREVENTING CARDIOVASCULAR DISEASE

Cardiovascular Complications In Diabetes

Diabetes is a particularly malicious metabolic disorder. Circulatory problems and clogging can occur in virtually every part of the 60,000-mile-long vessel pipeline.

Frequent Cardiovascular Complications In Diabetic Patients:

- Blindness from clogging of the arteries of the eyes
- Kidney failure from clogging of the kidney arteries, requiring dialysis
- Gangrene from clogging of the small arteries of the toes
- Heart attacks from clogging of the coronary arteries
- Strokes from clogging of brain arteries

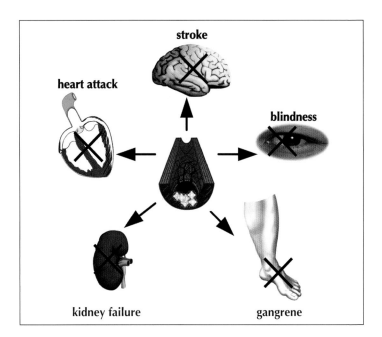

CARDIOVASCULAR COMPLICATIONS CAN OCCUR ANYWHERE IN THE BODY OF A DIABETIC

Vitamins and Diabetic Condition

Clinical studies show that vitamin C in diabetic patients not only contributes to prevention of cardiovascular complications but also helps to normalize the imbalance in the glucose metabolism. Professor R. Pfleger and his colleagues from the University of Vienna published the results of a remarkable clinical study. They showed that diabetic patients taking 300 to 500 mg of vitamin C a day could significantly improve glucose balance. Blood sugar levels could be lowered on average by 30%, daily insulin requirements by 27%, and sugar excretion in the urine could be almost eliminated. It is amazing that this study was published in 1937 in a leading European journal for internal medicine. If the results of this important study had been followed up and documented in medical textbooks, millions of lives would have been saved and cardiovascular disease would no longer threaten diabetic patients.

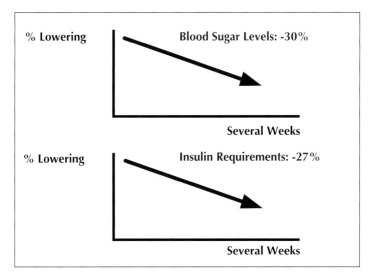

CLINICAL STUDY IN DIABETIC PATIENTS SHOWS: VITAMIN C LOWERS BLOOD SUGAR LEVELS AND INSULIN REQUIREMENT

Study Shows: the More Vitamin C, the Less Insulin

Diabetic patients can significantly lower their daily insulin requirements by increasing their daily intake of vitamin C. This is the result of a clinical case study conducted at the renowned Stanford University in California. Dr. J.F. Dice, the lead author of the study, was the diabetic patient of this case report.

At the beginning of the study Dr. Dice injected 32 units of insulin per day. During the three-week study, he gradually increased the daily intake of vitamin C until he reached 11 grams per day on the 23rd day. The vitamin C was divided in small amounts and taken throughout the day to increase its absorption in the body. By the 23rd day, his insulin requirement had dropped from 32 units to 5 units per day. Thus, for every additional gram of dietary vitamin C supplementation, Dr. Dice could spare about 2 units of insulin.

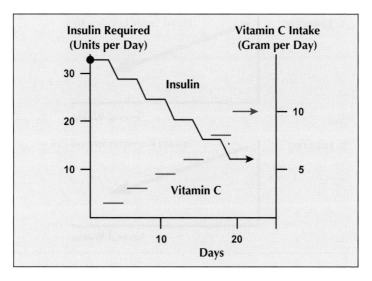

CLINICAL STUDY SHOWS: EACH ADDITIONAL GRAM OF VITAMIN C CAN SPARE ABOUT 2 UNITS OF INSULIN

Benefits of Vitamins in Diabetic Patients

The following sequence documents a selection of letters from patients with diabetic disorders. I encourage you to share these letters and the contents of this book with anyone you know suffering from diabetes. By doing so, you can help prevent heart attacks, strokes, blindness, and other organ failure in these patients.

Dear Dr. Rath,
I started ftaking the vitamin program three months ago. **I'm 29 years old and was recently diagnosed with Type II Diabetes. Since following your program on a regular basis, I have found my blood glucose level to remain around 100, even when under stress, which previously raised my blood glucose level.**

This vitamin program and 1-2 extra grams of vitamin C have relieved the primary negative symptoms that I have experienced

Sincerely, A.M.

Other Clinical Studies

Different nutrients have been shown in clinical studies to have health benefits for diabetic patients:

Nutrient	References
Vitamin C	Mann, Som, Stankova, Stepp
Vitamin E	Paolisso
Magnesium	McNair, Mather
Chromium	Liu, Riales

Nutrients Important in Diabetes

The following cellular bioenergy factors *in addition to* regular medication are important in diabetic conditions:

- Vitamin C: corrects the cellular imbalance caused by elevated blood sugar levels, contributes to lower insulin requirements, decreases glucose elimination in the urine and, above all, protects the artery walls.

- Vitamin E: anti-oxidant protection, protection of the cell membranes.

- Vitamin B1, B2, B3, B5, B6, B12 and Biotin: bioenergy carriers of cellular metabolism, improved metabolic efficacy, particularly of the liver cells, the central unit of the body metabolism.

- Chromium: trace element, functioning as a bio-catalyst for optimum metabolism of glucose and insulin.

- Inositol: component of lecithin, an important component of each cell membrane, essential for optimum metabolic transport and supply of each cell with nutrients and other bio molecules.

- Choline: component of lecithin, important for the metabolic transport and cellular supply of millions of cells.

Please note: the most important goal is to provide optimum protection for your artery walls, not to completely substitute for your insulin. In many cases, particularly in patients with inherited (juvenile) insulin deficiency, substituting vitamins for insulin will not be possible. Always consult with your doctor.

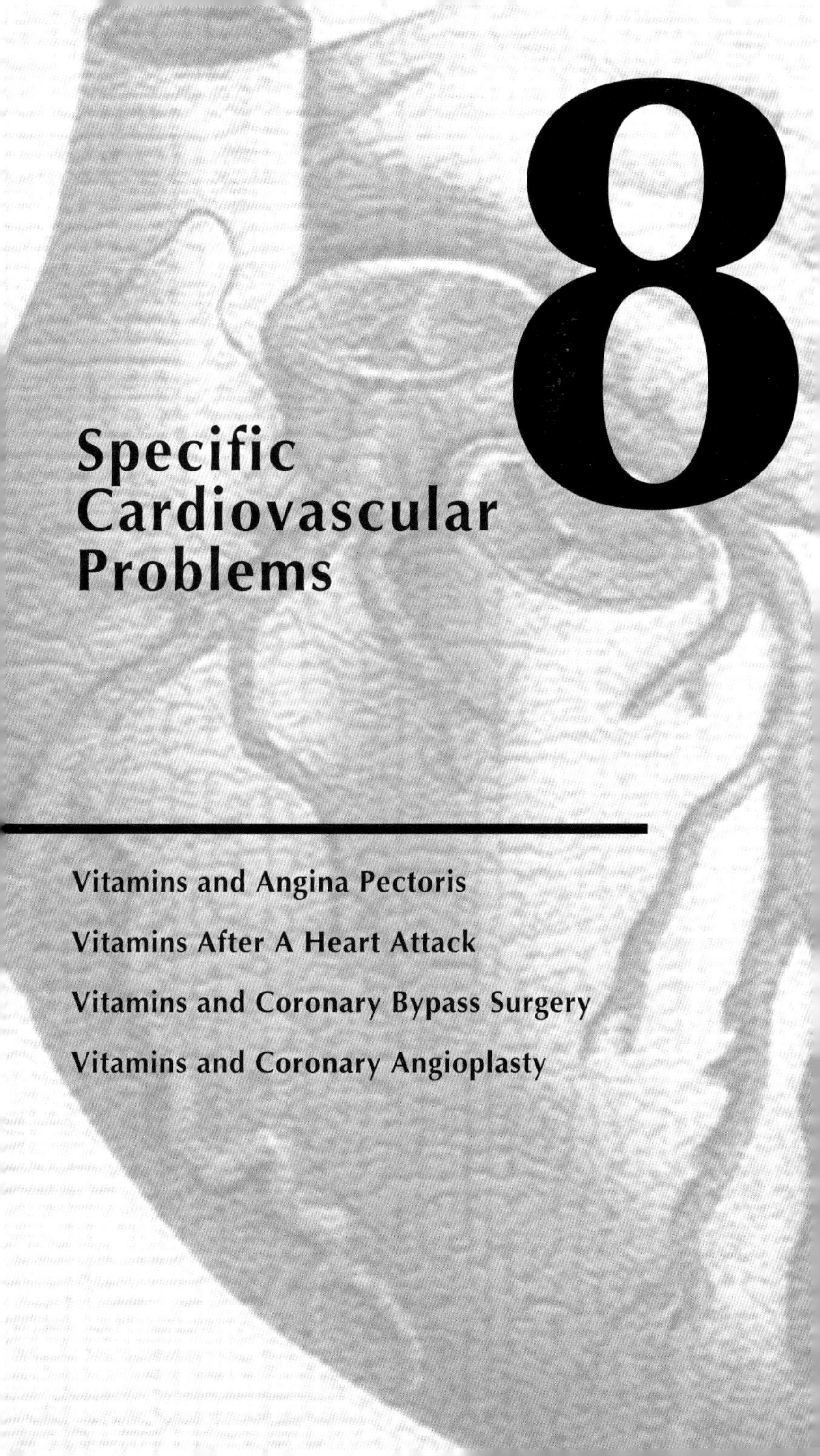

8

Specific Cardiovascular Problems

Vitamins and Angina Pectoris

Vitamins After A Heart Attack

Vitamins and Coronary Bypass Surgery

Vitamins and Coronary Angioplasty

Vitamins and Angina Pectoris

Angina pectoris is the typical alarm signal for atherosclerotic deposits in the coronary arteries. Angina pectoris is typically a sharp pain in the middle of the chest which frequently radiates into the left arm. Because there are many atypical forms of angina pectoris, I advise you to consult a physician about any form of chest pain.

Vitamins and other nutrients can help to improve the blood supply to the heart muscle cells by providing oxygen and nutrients, thereby decreasing angina pectoris. Several essential nutrients work together to achieve this aim. The most important ingredients are the following:

- Optimum supply of vitamin C and magnesium, as well as the natural amino acid, arginine, to aid widening of the coronary arteries and thereby increasing blood through the coronary arteries to the heart muscle cells.

- Carnitine, coenzyme Q10, B vitamins, certain minerals, and trace elements improve the performance of the heart muscle cells, the pumping function of the heart, the pressure by which the blood is pumped through the coronary arteries and, thereby, the supply of oxygen and nutrients to the heart muscle cells.

- Over a period of many months, vitamin C, lysine and proline initiate the healing process of the artery walls and the decrease of atherosclerotic deposits by the mechanisms described in detail earlier in this book.

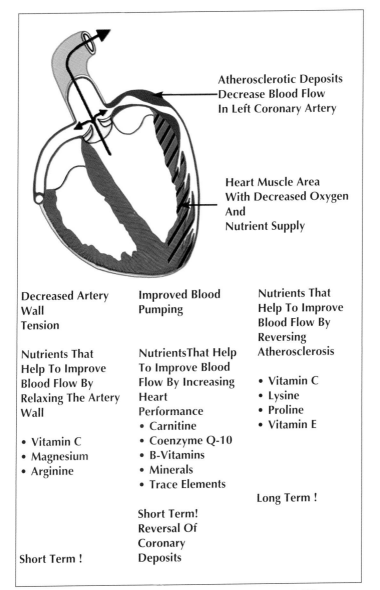

Atherosclerotic Deposits
Decrease Blood Flow
In Left Coronary Artery

Heart Muscle Area
With Decreased Oxygen
And
Nutrient Supply

Decreased Artery Wall Tension

Nutrients That Help To Improve Blood Flow By Relaxing The Artery Wall

• Vitamin C
• Magnesium
• Arginine

Short Term !

Improved Blood Pumping

NutrientsThat Help To Improve Blood Flow By Increasing Heart Performance
• Carnitine
• Coenzyme Q-10
• B-Vitamins
• Minerals
• Trace Elements

**Short Term!
Reversal Of Coronary Deposits**

Nutrients That Help To Improve Blood Flow By Reversing Atherosclerosis

• Vitamin C
• Lysine
• Proline
• Vitamin E

Long Term !

VITAMIN PROGRAMS AND OTHER NUTRIENTS HELP TO DECREASE AND PREVENT ANGINA PECTORIS

Benefits of Vitamins and Other Nutrients in Angina Pectoris

The following is a selection of letters from patients with coronary artery disease and angina pectoris. They document the benefits of natural vitamin programs so angina pectoris patients around the world can take advantage of this medical breakthrough and improve their quality of life.

Dear Dr. Rath,

I am so happy to tell you of the use of your vitamin program and how I feel that it has saved my life. Last September I had gone to the university to watch a football game and could not make it up the steps in the stadium despite wearing a nitroglycerin patch, and **by October last year I could not walk 100 yards without the pain of angina.**

I found out about your discovery and took it triple strength four times a day for three weeks and by Thanksgiving I had forgotten I had a heart problem. Now, in July of this year I am working without pain and feeling super!

Too bad you did not have the patent before I had undergone two bypass surgeries.

Thanks for more life, J.G.

Dear Dr. Rath:

I started taking vitamins last August after I was diagnosed as having severe heart disease. **I had angina for 8 years. Now, nearly a year later, I feel fine and have very slight angina infrequently, plus I walk 3.6 miles daily and don't have any restrictions.**

Sincerely, M.B

Clinical Studies With Nutrients In Angina Pectoris

An increasing number of clinical studies with various vitamins and other nutrients confirm that a decrease of angina pectoris is possible with supplementation of these essential nutrients. The following table summarizes some of the most important of these clinical studies:

Nutrient	References
Vitamin C, Vitamin E	Riemersma
Beta carotene	Riemersma
Carnitine	Ferrari, Opie
Coenzyme Q10	Folkers, Kamikawa
Magnesium	Iseri, Teo

The Consequences of a Heart Attack for the Body

A heart attack is caused by complete clogging of a coronary artery and by preventing oxygen and other nutrients from reaching heart muscle cells. Two main complications generally result from a heart attack:

- **Impaired pumping function (heart failure):** The area of the heart muscle that died weakens heart pumping. This results in impaired circulation, shortness of breath, edema, and severe fatigue. The effect of the failure of 25% of the heart muscles after a heart attack is like a four-cylinder motor running on three cylinders.

- **Impaired electrical conduction (irregular heartbeat):** In a similar way, the electrical cells of the heart can be affected by a heart attack. This can lead to various forms of irregular heart beat. Severe forms of arrhythmia are the most frequent causes of death after a heart attack.

117

How Vitamins and Other Nutrients Can Improve Quality Of Life After A Heart Attack

Anybody suffering a heart attack should be transported imme-diately to the nearest hospital. The sooner a patient receives proper medical attention, the greater the chance of limiting the lasting damage to the heart muscle cells. If a heart attack occurred some time ago, you should continue to consult regu-larly with your physician. In addition, a vitamin program can help in the following way to improve the quality of life:

- **Halting the development of atherosclerotic deposits** in the coronary arteries, thereby helping to prevent further heart attacks. The most important nutrients are vitamin C and other antioxidant vitamins, as well as the amino acids lysine and proline.

- **Optimizing the function of heart muscle cells still alive.** This is particularly important in the heart muscle area immedi-ately bordering the dead heart muscle area, where millions of cells are functioning at an impaired level. The most impor-tant nutrients are the B vitamins, carnitine, coenzyme Q10, as well as many minerals and trace elements.

Thus, it is not surprising that heart attack patients who start taking vitamins and other essential nutrients for optimum cardiovascular health experience significant health improvements.

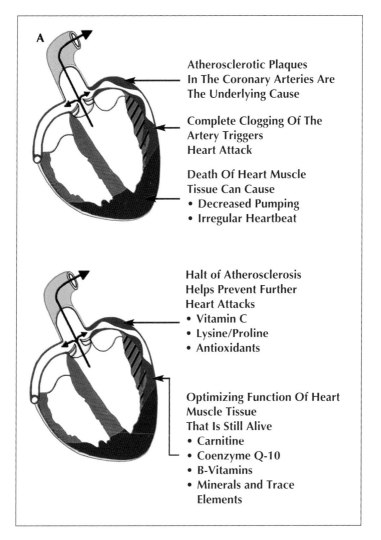

A: The Consequences of a Heart Attack

B: How Vitamin Program Contributes To An Improved Quality Of Life After A Heart Attack

Vitamins And Coronary Bypass Surgery

What Is a Coronary Bypass Operation?

A coronary bypass operation becomes necessary if one or more coronary arteries have developed severe atherosclerotic deposits that threaten to clog the arteries and to cause a heart attack. It surgically constructs a bypass around the atherosclerotic deposits in order to guarantee unrestricted blood flow to all parts of the heart muscle.

During a bypass operation, a vein is generally taken from the leg and re-implanted as a bypass blood vessel. One end of the bypass is attached to the aorta and the other end to the coronary artery beyond the location narrowed by an atherosclerotic deposit. Other bypass surgery procedures use smaller arteries in the vicinity of the heart to construct a bypass and to improve blood supply to the heart muscle.

I am often asked whether a coronary bypass operation can be avoided by supplementing with a vitamin program. As documented in this book, the operation can, in many cases, be postponed or cancelled. However, in other cases the atherosclerotic deposits have grown so far that a bypass operation is unavoidable. In any case, the decision can only be made together with your cardiologist. But even if a bypass operation has become inevitable, the vitamin supplementation can improve the long-term success of this operation and prevent further damage.

What Are the Main Problems After a Coronary Bypass Operation?

The overall success of a coronary artery bypass operation is threatened by two main problems:

- **Blood clots.** Blood clots can form in the bypass blood vessels, cutting off the blood flow. This complication normally occurs immediately after the operation. If untreated, this blood clot will completely cut off the blood flow through the bypass blood vessel and thereby make the previous operation ineffective.

- **Atherosclerotic deposits.** The greatest threat to the long-term success of a coronary bypass operation is the development of atherosclerotic deposits in the newly implanted bypass blood vessels. Although the bypass blood vessel is generally a vein, lesions and cracks can develop if they are not prevented by an optimum intake of vitamins and other essential nutrients. This triggers atherosclerotic deposits similar to those in the coronary arteries and, can eventually require a second bypass operation.

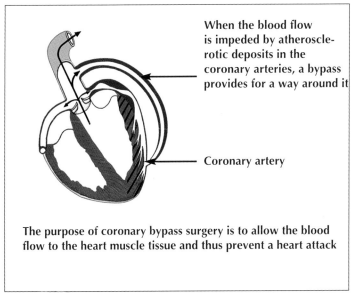

When the blood flow is impeded by atherosclerotic deposits in the coronary arteries, a bypass provides for a way around it

Coronary artery

The purpose of coronary bypass surgery is to allow the blood flow to the heart muscle tissue and thus prevent a heart attack

WHY BYPASS SURGERY IS PERFORMED

The Long-Term Success Of Coronary Bypass Surgery

There are several ways in which nutritional supplements help to maintain healthy bypass blood vessels and thereby improve the quality of life after bypass surgery.

• **Preventing blood clot formation in bypass blood vessels.** Vitamin C, vitamin E, and beta carotene have all been shown to help prevent the formation of blood clots. Vitamin C has also been shown to help dissolve existing blood clots. Patients on Coumadin and other "blood thinners" should inform their doctors when they start taking supplemental nutrients so that additional tests for blood coagulation can be done and less blood-thinning medication may be prescribed.

• **Preventing atherosclerotic deposits in bypass blood vessels.** The vitamins and other essential nutrients recommended for the prevention and adjunct reversal of atherosclerotic deposits in coronary arteries are also beneficial for preventing the development of atherosclerotic deposits in bypass blood vessels. The most important among these essential nutrients are vitamin C, vitamin E, beta-carotene, and the amino acids lysine and proline.

If you are scheduled for a bypass operation, I recommend that you start with this vitamin program as soon as possible. In this way, you make sure that the cells of the heart, the blood vessels, and other body tissues already hold an optimum level of vitamins and other bioenergy molecules during and imme-diately after the operation. This is the best way to optimize the healing process naturally (see also chapter 9).

1. Complication: **Blood Clot Formation In Bypass Vessels:**

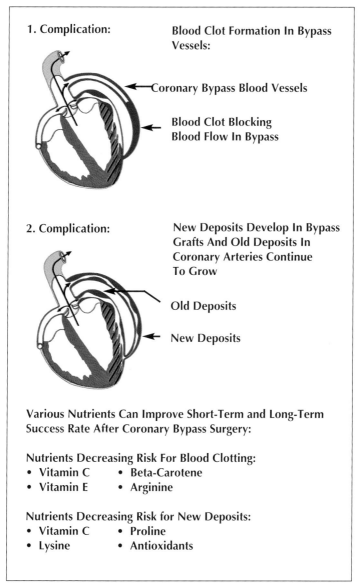

←Coronary Bypass Blood Vessels

←Blood Clot Blocking Blood Flow In Bypass

2. Complication: **New Deposits Develop In Bypass Grafts And Old Deposits In Coronary Arteries Continue To Grow**

Old Deposits

←New Deposits

Various Nutrients Can Improve Short-Term and Long-Term Success Rate After Coronary Bypass Surgery:

Nutrients Decreasing Risk For Blood Clotting:
- Vitamin C
- Vitamin E
- Beta-Carotene
- Arginine

Nutrients Decreasing Risk for New Deposits:
- Vitamin C
- Lysine
- Proline
- Antioxidants

OBSTACLES TO THE LONG-TERM SUCCESS OF CORONARY BYPASS SURGERY AND HOW VITAMIN PROGRAM HELPS TO PREVENT THEM

How Vitamins Improve the Long-Term Results of Coronary Angioplasty

What Is a Coronary Angioplasty?

In contrast to coronary bypass surgery, coronary angioplasty is the "Roto-Rooter" approach to removing atherosclerotic deposits. This approach generally involves an inflatable balloon or, more recently, laser or scraping methods. Generally, a catheter is inserted into the leg artery and moved forward through the aorta until the catheter tip reaches the coronary artery close to the deposits. At this point, a balloon at the tip of the catheter is inflated with high pressure, thereby squeezing the atherosclerotic deposits flat against the wall of the arteries. In many cases, the blood flow through the coronary artery can be improved by this procedure.

All angioplasty procedures damage the inside of the coronary arteries, sometimes over a distance of several inches. It is, therefore, not surprising that the rate of complications of this procedure is sobering. In over 30% of cases, a restenosis occurs, leading to the clogging of the coronary artery within as short a time as six months.

The most dangerous complication during the procedure is the rupturing of the wall of the coronary artery, requiring immediate bypass operation. Following the procedure, blood clots and small pieces of artery wall tissue can lead to a clogging of the coronary artery. Long-term complications include the overgrowth of scar tissue inside the coronary artery and the continued development of atherosclerotic deposits.

A good vitamin program can help patients scheduled for coronary angioplasty in different ways. In some cases, it can help decrease angina pectoris and other signs of coronary heart disease enough that your doctor will suggest postponement of the angioplasty procedure. In other cases, your doctor will advise you to carry out the procedure to minimize your risk of a heart attack. In any case, you should follow the advice of your doctor. At the same time, I recommend that you start this vitamin program as soon as possible and inform your doctor about it. If you have already undergone coronary angioplasty,

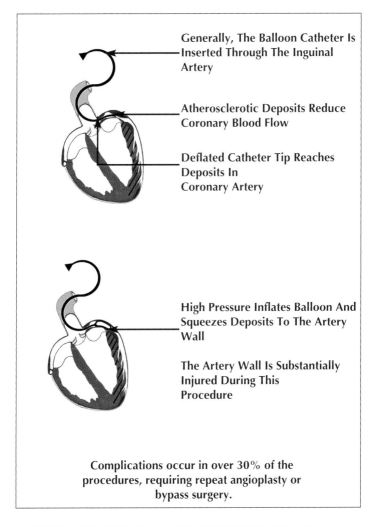

Generally, The Balloon Catheter Is Inserted Through The Inguinal Artery

Atherosclerotic Deposits Reduce Coronary Blood Flow

Deflated Catheter Tip Reaches Deposits In Coronary Artery

High Pressure Inflates Balloon And Squeezes Deposits To The Artery Wall

The Artery Wall Is Substantially Injured During This Procedure

Complications occur in over 30% of the procedures, requiring repeat angioplasty or bypass surgery.

ANGIOPLASTY INEVITABLY CAUSES SUBSTANTIAL DAMAGE TO THE ARTERY WALL

Dr. Rath's Vitamin Program can help you to improve the long-term success of this procedure.

- Vitamin C accelerates healing of the wounds in the coronary arteries caused by the angioplasty procedure.

- Lysine and proline help in the re-formation of the artery wall and at the same time decrease the risk of fatty deposits.

- Vitamin E and vitamin C help control excessive scar tissue from the uncontrolled growth of arterial wall muscle cells.

- Vitamin C, vitamin E, and beta-carotene decrease the risk of blood clot formation and provide important antioxidant protection.

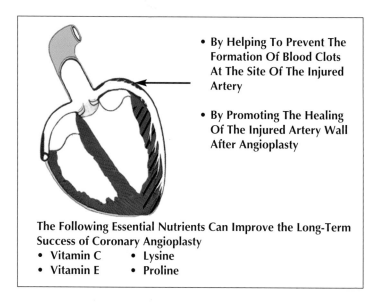

- **By Helping To Prevent The Formation Of Blood Clots At The Site Of The Injured Artery**

- **By Promoting The Healing Of The Injured Artery Wall After Angioplasty**

The Following Essential Nutrients Can Improve the Long-Term Success of Coronary Angioplasty
- **Vitamin C**   • **Lysine**
- **Vitamin E**   • **Proline**

VITAMINS CAN IMPROVE THE SUCCESS RATE OF CORONARY ANGIOPLASTY

Further Health Information Related to Essential Nutrients and Angioplasty

Research and clinical studies have confirmed the important role of different nutrients in decreasing the risk of clogging of coronary arteries after angioplasty:

Dr. S.J. DeMeio from Emory University in Atlanta, Georgia, U.S.A., studied patients with coronary heart disease who underwent coronary angioplasty. After this procedure, one group of the patients received 1,200 International Units (I.U.) of vitamin E as a nutritional supplement. The control group received no additional vitamin E. After four months, the patients who had received vitamin E showed a 15% decrease in the rate of coronary restenosis compared to those patients without vitamin E supplementation.

My colleague, Dr. Aleksandra Niedzwiecki, and her collaborators showed that vitamin C decreases the overgrowth of the smooth muscle cells of the artery wall and thereby helps to control one of the most frequent factors responsible for the failure of angioplasty procedures. Animal experiments by Dr. G.L. Nunes and his colleagues confirmed these observations for vitamin C and vitamin E.

The benefit of a vitamin program over the use of single nutrients is that it contains a selection of essential nutrients that work synergistically to improve the long-term success after coronary angioplasty. Of course, you can also increase the amounts of specific vitamins, such as vitamin C and vitamin E, to further enhance this effect.

9

External and Inherited Cardiovascular Risks

- Unhealthy Diet
- Smoking
- Stress
- Hormonal Contraceptives
- Diuretic Medication
- Other Prescription Drugs
- Dialysis
- Surgery
- Inherited Cardiovascular Risk Factors

Unhealthy Diet

The basis of any natural cardiovascular health program is a healthy diet. For many generations, the diet of our ancestors shaped the metabolism of our bodies. By understanding our ancestors' diet, we have learned what is best for our bodies today. Their diet was rich in grains, fruits, vegetables, and other plant nutrition high in fiber and vitamins. They ate considerably less fat and sugar than we do today. In contrast, the average diet in the industrialized countries imposes a heavy metabolic burden on our bodies. Certain inherited disorders put our bodies at further risk. Thus, it is good to know that many specific nutrients have been shown to optimize our metabolism. This is particularly important for the metabolism of fat in our body.

This vitamin program helps you to:

- Lower cholesterol production in the body
- Optimize the metabolism of fat molecules in cells
- Optimize the elimination of fat from the body
- Protect fat molecules from oxidation

It is important to understand that certain vitamins are used in the degradation process of these fat molecules. For example, for every molecule of cholesterol, whether it is produced in the body or comes from the diet, our body consumes one molecule of vitamin C in an enzymatic reaction in the liver. In this way, high cholesterol and triglyceride levels can contribute to a chronic vitamin depletion of the body. Thus, it is important to understand that the increased cardiovascular risk is not primarily the result of too many fat molecules in the diet, but it comes from the systematic depletion of the vitamin reserves in our bodies from an overburdened fat metabolism. As a consequence of chronic vitamin depletion, the artery walls are weakened and cardiovascular disease develops.

Besides too much fat, there are other dangers in our diet. Residues from herbicides, pesticides, and chemical preservatives are present in every meal we eat. These toxic substances have to be detoxified in our liver. Vitamin C and other vitamins, minerals and trace elements are essential cofactors for a rapid detoxification of these substances in our bodies.

My recommendation

Eat a prudent diet. Watch your weight, and exercise regularly. As a general rule, a healthy diet is:
• rich in natural foods: plant nutrition, fish, lean meat
• low in processed foods and artificial foods

More specifically, you should eat a diet:
• rich in natural fiber (complex carbohydrates)
• rich in vitamins
• low in sugars (sweeteners)
• moderate amounts of fats

Why is this nutrition recommended? This is the nutrition our ancestors have had over thousands of generations. These dietary principles have shaped our digestive system and the proper function of the human body over millennia. This is why our body today is responding favorably to these nutritional principles.

There are some health gurus who try to promote one or another ingredient in our diet; for example, a minimum fat diet or a minimum carbohydrate diet. There is no scientific basis for omitting entire groups of macronutrients (fat, proteins or carbohydrates) from our diet.

The only scientific basis for a prudent diet for you is to understand the principles of the diet our ancestors followed for thousands of years (see above) and to adapt those principles to our modern diet. In addition, supplement your diet (macronutrients) with vitamins and other micronutrients.

Smoking

While it is generally known that smoking dramatically increases the risk for cardiovascular disease, the underlying reason is unclear. The smoke from cigarettes contains millions of free radicals, those aggressive molecules that damage the cells of our body organs and accelerate the biological rusting. Free radicals and other toxic substances in cigarette smoke reach the blood stream from the lungs. These noxious substances can damage the blood vessel pipeline along its entire length of 60,000 miles. Now we understand why smokers have a specific form of atherosclerosis, which frequently starts in the body periphery, e.g., the toes, feet, and legs. In this case, atherosclerosis is not limited to the coronary arteries, but the damage also occurs in the small arteries and capillaries throughout the body. The "smoker foot" is proverbial and often toes, the foot, or part of the leg must be amputated.

My recommendation is

If you still smoke, it is worth every effort to stop. Perhaps this chapter will help you become aware of how much damage you actually cause in your body by smoking. For smokers and ex-smokers, my recommendations are the same: Optimize your daily intake of natural antioxidants, preferably in the form of a vitamin and essential nutrient program.

Stress

Chronic physical and psychological stress increase the risk for cardiovascular disease. What is the underlying biochemical mechanism for this phenomenon? During physical or emotional stress, the body produces high amounts of the stress hormone adrenaline. For every molecule of adrenaline produced, the body needs a molecule of vitamin C as the catalyst. These vitamin C molecules are destroyed in these reactions. Thus, long-term physical or emotional stress can lead to a severe depletion of the body's reservoir of vitamin C. If vitamin C is not supplemented in the diet, the cardiovascular system is weakened, and atherosclerosis develops.

These facts also explain why spouses frequently die soon after one another. The loss of a partner results in long-term emotional stress and a rapid vitamin depletion of the body, thereby increasing the risk for a heart attack. We have to understand that it is not the emotional stress itself that causes the heart attack, but the biochemical consequence.

My recommendation is

Find time to relax. Schedule hours and days to relax just as you schedule your professional appointments. With severe emotional problems, you may also benefit from professional consultation. Irrespective of these steps, make sure that you supplement your body's reservoir of vitamins and other nutrients in the form of a vitamin program.

Hormonal Contraceptives

Several studies show that women taking hormonal contraceptives ("The Pill") significantly increase their risk for cardiovascular disease. What is the biochemical basis for this phenomenon? In 1972, Dr. M. Briggs reported in the scientific journal, *Nature*, that women taking hormonal contraceptives had significantly lower vitamin C blood levels than normal. In another study, Dr. J.M. Rivers confirmed these results and concluded that the vitamin C depletion is associated with the estrogen hormone. The fact is that long-term use of hormone contraceptives decreases the body pool of vitamin C and also of other essential nutrients. Thus, it is not the birth control pill itself that increases the risk for cardiovascular disease, but the associated depletion of the body's vitamin pool, leading to a weakening of the blood vessel wall.

My recommendation is

If you are taking hormonal birth control pills, or if you have taken them in the past, I recommend that you start following vitamin programs to resupply your body's vitamin pool and to prevent its future depletion.

Diuretic Drugs

Taking diuretic drugs can significantly increase your risk for cardiovascular disease. Diuretics flush not only water from the body but also water soluble vitamins and other essential nutrients. I described this mechanism in detail in the chapter on Heart Failure. The importance of a regular supplementation of these vitamins and other essential nutrients in patients taking diuretics cannot be over emphasized.

Other Prescription Drugs

Besides diuretics, all prescription drugs currently taken by millions of people lead to a gradual depletion of vitamins and other components of a vitamin program in the body. Drugs are generally synthetic, non-natural substances. Different drugs can contribute in different ways to the depletion of the body's vitamin reserves:

All synthetic drugs have to be detoxified by the liver in order to be eliminated from the body. This detoxification process requires vitamin C and other vitamins and nutrients as cofactors. Many of these essential nutrients are used up in biocatalytic reactions during this "detoxification" process. Thus, long-term use of many synthetic prescription drugs leads to a chronic vitamin depletion of the body and, thereby, to the onset of cardiovascular disease. Another way in which prescription drugs, such as the cholesterol-lowering agent Cholestyramine, contribute to vitamin depletion is their binding to vitamins in the digestive tract. This prevents optimum absorption of vitamins from the digestive tract into the bloodstream and the body.

Prescription drugs can also deplete the body's reservoir of certain essential nutrients by interfering with the natural production of these essential nutrients. For instance, cholesterol-lowering drugs of the "statin" group inhibit the production of cholesterol in the cells of the body. Unfortunately, they also decrease the production of important natural molecules in the body, such as coenzyme Q10 (ubiquinone). Professor K. Folkers, from the University of Texas in Austin, reported that heart failure patients with low baseline coenzyme Q10 levels can experience life-threatening cardiovascular complications when taking these cholesterol-lowering drugs because of a further decrease of coenzyme Q10 in the body.

My recommendation is

If you are taking any prescription drug, I recommend that you also begin taking a vitamin program. Play it safe. Follow the recommendations of this book, and inform your doctor about it.

Dialysis

Several investigations have shown that patients undergoing long-term dialysis have an increased risk of cardiovascular disease. This is not surprising, since dialysis eliminates not only the body's waste products from the blood but also many vitamins and other essential nutrients. If these essential nutrients are not restored, chronic dialysis will lead to a gradual depletion of vitamins and other essential nutrients throughout the body, thereby triggering atherosclerosis and cardiovascular disease.

My recommendation is

If you are undergoing dialysis, you should immediately start a comprehensive vitamin and mineral program. If you know a dialysis patient, please make sure that you hand over the information from this book; you could help prolong a life.

Surgery

Patients undergoing an operation should make sure that the cells of their bodies are optimally supplied with vitamins and other essential nutrients. This can help you before, during, and after the operation. Such a vitamin program should help replace the essential nutrients depleted during the physical and emotional stress of an operation. Each operation results in extraordinary physical and psychological stress for the patient.

I have already explained the direct connection between stress and vitamin depletion. Preparation for the operation, the procedure itself, and the healing phase after an operation frequently results in high stress for several weeks, and can lead to a serious vitamin depletion of your body at a time of great need.

Each operation is associated with damage to body tissue to a lesser or greater extent. The speed at which the operation wound heals is directly related to the rate at which collagen and other connective tissue molecules are formed and heal the wound. Vitamins and other nutrients can help to accelerate wound healing.Vitamin C and other essential nutrients are your best natural options for optimizing the production of collagen molecules and to speed up the healing phase after an operation.

Antioxidant nutrients are important in protecting against oxidative damage during operations. A variety of operation procedures require an extra-corporeal circulation during the operation itself. During a bypass operation, for example, the heartbeat is artificially stopped and the blood circulation is maintained by a heart-lung machine. During this extra-corporeal circulation, the patient's blood is artificially enriched with oxygen. It is a well known fact that high concentrations of oxygen can lead to tissue damage of the artery walls and other body tissues (reperfusion injury). Antioxidants can minimize the risks of oxidative damage during an operation.

These are the reasons why every patient should start on antioxidants as soon as possible before an operation. Inform your doctor about it and follow a vitamin program while in the hospital. If your doctors are still reluctant to approve this program, you can tell them that Harvard Medical School and other leading medical universities are now routinely recommending vitamin supplementation to their patients undergoing surgery.

The following table summarizes some of the studies underlining the importance of vitamins and other nutrients in decreasing different external risk factors for cardiovascular disease:

External Risk Factors Studied	References
Blood Fats	Ginter, Harwood, Sokoloff
Smoking	Chow, Halliwell, Lehr, Riemersma
Stress	Levine
"The Pill"	Briggs, Rivers
Dialysis	Blumberg
Prescription Drugs	Halliwell, Clemetson

Patients with the following inherited disorders should consider following the vitamin program in addition to their regular treatment should inform their doctors about it.

– **Diabetes**
– **Homocystinuria**
– **Alzheimer's Disease**
– **Neurofibromatosis**
– **Cystic Fibrosis**
– **Lupus Erythematosus**
– **Scleroderma**
– **Muscular Dystrophy**
– **Parkinson's Disease**
– **Multiple Sclerosis**
– **Addison's Disease**
– **Amyloidosis**
– **Morbus Cushing**
– **Down's Syndrome**
– **Rheumatoid Arthritis**
– **Connective Tissue Disorders**

Inherited Cardiovascular Risk Factors

I am frequently asked whether the vitamin program can also help decrease the risk of inherited risk factors. In many cases, the answer is "yes." Besides the external risk factors discussed in the previous section, inherited, or genetic, risk is the second largest group of cardiovascular risk factors. We have all heard the sentence, "Heart disease runs in our family." Members of these families frequently die in the fourth or fifth decade of their lives. The causes of these early deaths are, at least in part, caused by abnormal genes (molecules of inheritance), which are passed on from generation to generation in that family. Earlier in this book I described two of the most frequent genetic risk factors – inherited disorders of fat metabolism (high cholesterol, hypercholesterolemia) and inherited disorders of sugar metabolism (diabetes).

It is important to understand that this genetic risk is no death sentence. The genetic deficiency generally results in an impaired metabolic function at one location or another in our cellular software program (see first chapters of this book). In most cases, this genetic impairment can be compensated for by an increased intake of essential nutrients. As we already know, vitamins and other essential nutrients are cellular energy carriers and they are able to speed up biochemical reactions that are impaired.

It is therefore no surprise that vitamins and other essential nutrients have already been shown to have profound health benefits in patients with genetic disorders.

The table left provides a list of inherited disorders. Patients with these disorders can benefit from nutrient supplementation.

If you know anyone with one of the inherited diseases listed in the table, please introduce this information to them. As you can see from the history of the Alzheimer's and lupus erythematosus patients at the end of this section, these patients can only win by immediately starting Dr. Rath's Vitamin Program, a natural and safe approach to these health conditions. This is even more important considering the fact that conventional medicine has no answers to these serious health problems.

How do vitamins and other nutrients lessen the cardiovascular risk associated with these inherited risk factors? Let's take diabetes, for example. With this disease, a genetic defect produces an insufficient amount of the insulin hormone. The clinical consequences are discussed in detail in the diabetes chapter. Although a vitamin program cannot repair the defective gene, it can help prevent triggering of the diabetic glucose imbalance, as well as development of diabetic cardiovascular complications. In the adjacent figure, the defective gene is symbolized as a time bomb. The nutritional supplement program cannot make this time bomb disappear; however, it can contribute to defusing it and thereby prevent an explosion in the form of a metabolic imbalance or the initiation of disease symptoms. As documented in this book for diabetes, cholesterol disorders, Alzheimer's Disease, Lupus Erythematosus and other conditions, vitamins are the first effective therapeutic approach to reduce the risk from inherited disorders, particularly the development of cardiovascular complications.

The adjacent figure summarizes the main factors contributing to your personal cardiovascular risk. Inherited risk factors plus external risk factors determine your overall risk for cardiovascular disease by gradually depleting your body's reservoir of essential nutrients. Most internal and external risk factors are effectively neutralized by an optimum intake of vitamins and other essential nutrients. You can minimize your cardiovascular risk by two distinct measures: increasing your daily intake of essential nutrients and minimizing your external risk factors such as smoking and an unhealthy diet.

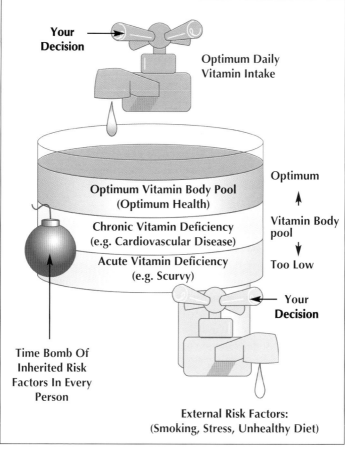

MAINTAINING AN OPTIMUM BODY POOL OF ESSENTIAL
NUTRIENTS IS THE KEY TO OPTIMUM HEALTH

Vitamins and Alzheimers Disease

Alzheimer's disease is a degenerative impairment of brain function. Conventional medicine has no therapy for this serious health problem.

Dear Dr. Rath:

My father, who is 84, has Alzheimer's Disease. About two months ago his caregivers attended an Alzheimer's seminar at a nursing home there. The seminar reported that some patients had been put on vitamin supplements, which had resulted in improved memory for several patients.

My father has been on the vitamin program for two months and we cannot believe the improvement. His short-term memory is improving and we can carry on conversations with him again. He is even showing some problem solving capabilities again. I know these improvements are not measurable from a "pure scientific perspective" but to us it's a blessing to see improvement rather than just deterioration from this terrible disease

On behalf of my father and our family, thank you for your research and information.
Yours truly, D.C.

Vitamin Program and Lupus Erythematosus

Lupus erythematosus is a so-called "autoimmune disease". It can lead to inflammation, hardening impairment, and eventually, failure of just about any organ in the body. Conventional medicine has no therapy for this serious health problem.

Dear Dr. Rath:

My sister suffered from lupus erythematosus disease. She was diagnosed with it in 1973 and since that time she has been hospitalized more times than I can remember and has **suffered from phlebitis (inflammation of the veins), shingles, ulcerative colitis (inflammation of the bowel), and her vision has steadily deteriorated.**

She is 44 years old, married and mother of 3 children. In 1989 a routine PAP-smear showed severe inflammation and pre-cancerous tissue. Her doctors tried to treat this condition with drugs first, and later with "laser burn" treatments. This reduced the number of cells somewhat but did not end the problem. A subsequent PAP-smear showed that the number of cells was increasing and they performed a complete hysterectomy. **Even after the hysterectomy she still had severe inflammation and a large number of pre-cancerous cells.**

Other treatments had been also ineffective. Basically, her doctors didn't know what else to try.

In November she began following the vitamin program. Even though she was somewhat skeptical, she felt that she had nothing to lose. After 8 months on your program she had another PAP-Smear test taken. What a tremendous feeling of joy she must have felt when her doctor told her that her PAP-smear came back **perfectly normal with no inflammation and no pre-cancerous cells.** Her doctor asked her what she was doing differently. She told her doctor about the vitamin program. Her doctor replied she didn't understand it, but couldn't argue with success.

There was also other benefit. When her ophthalmologist re-examined her eyes, the first thing he asked was: "What have you been doing differently since your previous check up?" **He said her eyes were "healthier" inside than he had ever seen them during the two and a half years he'd been treating her.**

Also, my sister is now able to limit her prednisone (anti-inflammatory medication) to the smallest dosage during the past 22 years.

Thank you for your research and for your efforts to spread the word of your breakthrough discovery.

Sincerely, S.S.

10

Cellular Health
And Vitamins

Vitamins and Other Nutrients As
Bioenergy Source

The Goal of Cellular Health

Scientific Facts About The Ingredients Of
Dr. Rath's Vitamin Program

Vitamin Programs Compared to
Conventional Therapies

Vitamins and Other Nutrients As Bioenergy Source

Vitamins and other nutrients are an essential part of the biological fuel we have to provide regularly to our bodies. The other biological fuels are well known: air (oxygen), water, macro-nutrients (composed of proteins, fats, and carbohydrates). A distinct characteristic separates vitamins from air, water, and food: a lack of vitamins and other essential nutrients does not give any alarm signs. Oxygen deficiency, for example, leads within minutes to suffocation. Water deficiency's alarm sign is thirst. Lack of food causes hunger.

In contrast, a deficiency of vitamins and other essential nutrients, gives no alarm signs. The first sign of a vitamin deficiency is the outbreak of a disease. A total depletion of vitamins, such as that in scurvy, leads to death within months. Since we all get small amounts of vitamins and other essential nutrients, we generally do not suffer from a total depletion.

Most of us, however, suffer from a chronic deficiency of vitamins and other essential nutrients. In many cases, the first sign of chronic vitamin deficiency is a heart attack or the outbreak of another disease. Thus, since our body does not give us any alarm signs, the best way we can avoid deficiencies in cellular energy is an optimum daily supplementation of essential vitamins and nutrients.

Oxygen	Water

Regular Food · Carbohydrates · Fat · Protein	**Essential Nutrients** · Vitamins · Amino Acids · Minerals · Trace elements

Missing Life Essentials		Early Alarm Signs		Death Occurs Within
No Oxygen	—	Suffocation	→	Minutes
No Water	—	Thirst	→	Days
No Food	—	Hunger	→	Weeks
Zero Vitamins	—	None !	→	Months (e.g. Scurvy)
Vitamin Deíciency	—	None !	→	Many Years (e.g. Heart Attack)

BIOENERGY SOURCES FOR THE BODY

Cellular Health

This book introduces the era of Cellular Health. This new era of health is based on a new understanding of wellness: Health and disease of our body is determined by the function of millions of cells. Optimum functioning of these building blocks of life means health; in contrast, cellular malfunction causes disease.

The primary cause of malfunctioning of cells is a chronic deficiency of essential nutrients, in particular of vitamins, amino acids, minerals, and trace elements. These essential nutrients are needed for a multitude of biochemical reactions and other cellular functions in every single cell of our body. Chronic deficiencies of one or more of these essential nutrients, therefore, must lead to cellular malfunctioning and to disease.

Cellular Health can also explain why cardiovascular disease is still the number one cause of death. The heart is the most active organ of our body because it continuously pumps blood through the circulatory system. Because of high mechanical demands, the cells of the cardiovascular system have a high rate of consumption of vitamins and other essential nutrients.

Finally, Cellular Health identifies an optimum daily intake of vitamins and other essential nutrients as a basic preventive and therapeutic measure for cardiovascular diseases as well as many other health conditions.

The Principles Of Cellular Health

I.   Health and disease are determined on the level of millions of cells which compose our body and its organs.

II. Vitamins and other essential nutrients are needed for thousands of biochemical reactions in each cell. Chronic deficiency of these vitamins and other essential nutrients is the most frequent cause of malfunction of millions of body cells and the primary cause of cardiovascular disease and other diseases.

III. Cardiovascular diseases are the most frequent diseases because cardiovascular cells consume vitamins and other essential nutrients at a high rate due to mechanical stress on the heart and the blood vessel wall from the heartbeat and the pulse wave.

IV. Optimum dietary supplementation of vitamins and other essential nutrients is the key to prevention and effective treatment of cardiovascular disease, as well as other chronic health conditions.

The Main Aim Of Cellular Health: Supply Of Cellular Energy

Most carriers of bioenergy in cellular metabolism are vitamins. The figure on page 151 summarizes important details:

- **Acetyl-Coenzyme A (Acetyl-CoA),** the central molecule of cellular metabolism, is indispensable for processing of all components of food (carbohydrates, proteins, fats) and for their conversion into bioenergy. Vitamin B5 (pantothenic acid) is a structural component of this key molecule. A deficiency of vitamin B5 leads to decreased Acetyl-Coenzyme A levels and to a metabolic "jam." This can result in increased levels of cholesterol and other blood fats. Optimum supplementation of vitamin B5 corrects this "jam" and improves the production of cellular energy.

- **Vitamin B3 (nicotinic acid)** is the energy transport molecule of one of the most important cellular energy carriers, called nicotinamide-adenine-dinucleotide (NAD). Vitamin C provides the bioenergy to the NAD transport molecules by adding hydrogen atoms (-H) and thereby, biological energy. The energy-rich shuttle molecules NAD-H provide energy for thousands of cellular reactions. Sufficient supply of vitamin B3 and vitamin C is indispensable for optimum cellular energy.

- **Vitamin B2 (riboflavin)** and vitamin C cooperate in a similar way within each cell as a bioenergy shuttle. Vitamin B2 is a structural component of the energy transport molecule flavin-adenine-dinucleotide (FAD) and vitamin C provides bioenergy for the activation of millions of bioenergy-rich FAD molecules.

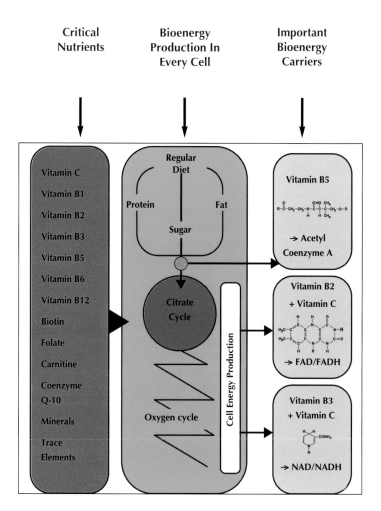

ESSENTIAL NUTRIENTS PROVIDE BIOENERGY FOR EACH CELL

Scientific Facts About the Health Benefits of Vitamins and Other Nutrients

Vitamins

Vitamin C
Vitamin C is the key nutrient for the stability of our blood vessels, our heart, and all other organs of our body. Without vitamin C our body would literally collapse and dissolve, as in scurvy.

Vitamin C is responsible for an optimum production and function of collagen, elastin and other connective tissue molecules that give stability to the blood vessel walls and to our body. Vitamin C is important for fast wound healing throughout our body, including the healing of millions of tiny wounds and lesions in the inside of our blood vessel walls.

Vitamin C is the most important antioxidant of the body. Optimum amounts of vitamin C protect the cardiovascular system and the body effectively against biological rusting.

Vitamin C is also a cofactor for a series of biological catalysts (enzymes) which are important for an improved metabolism of cholesterol, triglycerides and other risk factors. This helps to decrease the risk for cardiovascular disease.

Vitamin C is an important energy molecule to recharge energy carriers inside the cells.

Vitamin E
Vitamin E is the most important fat soluble antioxidant vitamin. It particularly protects the membranes of the cells in our cardiovascular system and our body against attacks from free radicals and against oxidative damage.

Vitamin E is enriched in low-density lipoproteins (LDL) and other cholesterol and fat transporting particles. Taken in optimum amounts, vitamin E can prevent these fat particles from oxidation (biological rusting) and from damaging the inside of the blood vessel walls.

Vitamin E was shown to render the platelets in our blood circulation less sticky, thereby keeping our blood thin and decreasing the risk from blood clotting.

Beta-Carotene
Beta-Carotene is also called pro-vitamin A and is another important fat soluble antioxidant vitamin. Like vitamin E, it is transported primarily in lipoprotein particles in our bloodstream to millions of body cells. Like vitamin E, beta-carotene protects these fat particles from rusting and from becoming damaging to the cardiovascular system. Considering these scientific facts, it is not surprising that vitamin C, vitamin E, and beta carotene are documented in a rapidly growing number of clinical studies as powerful protective agents against cardiovascular disease.

Similar to vitamin E, beta-carotene has been shown to decrease the risk of blood clotting.

Vitamin B-1 (Thiamin)
Thiamin functions as the cofactor for an important biocatalyst called pyrophosphate. This catalyst is involved in phosphate metabolism in our cells, another key energy source to optimize millions of reactions in our cardiovascular cells and our body.

Vitamin B-2 (Riboflavin)
Riboflavin is the cofactor for flavin-adenine-dinucleotide (FAD), one of the most important carrier molecules of cellular energy inside the tiny energy centers (power plants) of all cells.

Vitamin B-3 (Niacin, Niacinamide)
Niacin, an important nutrient, is a cofactor for nicotinamide-

155

adenine-dinucleotide (NAD) molecule. This energy carrier molecule is one of the most important energy transport systems in our entire body. Millions of these carriers are created and recharged (by vitamin C) inside the cellular energy centers of our cardiovascular system and our body. Cell life and life in general would not be possible without this energy carrier.

Vitamin B-5 (Pantothenate)
Pantothenate is the cofactor for coenzyme A, the central fuel molecule in the metabolism of our heart cells, our blood vessel cells and all other cells. The metabolism of carbohydrates, proteins and fats inside each cell lead into one single molecule, Acetyl Coenzyme A. This molecule is the key that helps convert all food into cell energy. It is actually composed in part of vitamin B-5, and the importance of supplementing with this vitamin is evident. Again, cell life would not be possible without this vitamin.

Vitamin B-6 (Pyridoxine)
Vitamin B-6 is the cofactor for pyridoxal phosphate, an important co-factor for the metabolism of amino acids and proteins in our cardiovascular cells and our body.

Vitamin B-6 is needed in the production of red blood cells, the carriers of oxygen to the cells of our cardiovascular system and all other cells of our body.

Vitamin B-6 is also essential for optimum structure and function of collagen fibers.

Vitamin B-12
Vitamin B-12 is needed for proper metabolism of fatty acids and certain amino acids in the cells of our body.

Vitamin B-12 is also required for the production of red blood cells. A severe deficiency of vitamin B-12 can cause pernicious anemia, characterized by an insufficient production of blood cells.

Folate
Folate is a very important nutrient for the production of red

blood cells and for oxygen supply.

The last three vitamins are good examples of how these bioenergy molecules work together like an orchestra. Without proper oxygen transport to all the cells, their function would be impaired, no matter how much of the other vitamins you take. It is therefore important to supplement your diet as completely as possible with the right essential nutrients in the right amounts.

Biotin
Biotin is needed in the metabolism of carbohydrates, fats and proteins.

Vitamin D
Vitamin D is essential for optimum calcium and phosphate metabolism in the body.

Vitamin D is indispensable for bone formation, growth, and stability of our skeleton. Over centuries, vitamin D deficiency was a frequent children's disease, causing retarded growth and malformation. Even today, milk is frequently supplemented with this vitamin.

In our body vitamin D can also be synthesized from cholesterol molecules by the action of light.

In connection with cardiovascular disease, Vitamin D is essential for optimum calcium metabolism in the artery walls, including the removal of calcium from atherosclerotic deposits.

Minerals

Minerals are important essential nutrients. Calcium, magnesium, and potassium are the most important among them. Minerals are needed for a multitude of catalytic reactions in each cell of our body.

Calcium

Calcium is important for the proper contraction of muscle cells, including millions of heart muscle cells.

Calcium is needed for conducting nerve impulses and an optimum heartbeat.

Calcium is also needed for the proper biological communication among the cells of the cardiovascular system and most other cells, as well as for many other biological functions.

Magnesium

Magnesium is nature's calcium antagonist, and its benefit for the cardiovascular system is similar to the calcium antagonist drugs that are prescribed, except that magnesium is produced by nature.

Clinical studies have shown that magnesium is particularly important for helping to normalize elevated blood pressure; moreover, it can help normalize irregular heartbeat.

Trace Elements

The trace elements zinc, manganese, copper, selenium, chromium, and molybdenum are also important essential nutrients. Most of them are metals needed as catalysts for thousands of reactions in the metabolism of cells. They are needed only in very tiny amounts – less than a tenth of a thousandth of a gram. Selenium is also a very important antioxidant.

Amino Acids

Amino acids are the building blocks of proteins. Most of the amino acids in our body are derived from regular food and from the breakdown of its protein content. Many amino acids can be synthesized in our body when needed; these are called "non-essential" amino acids. Those amino acids which the body cannot synthesize are called "essential" amino acids.

Interestingly, there is now important scientific evidence that even though the body can produce certain amino acids, the amount produced may not be enough to maintain proper health. A good example is the amino acid proline.

Proline

The amino acid proline is a major building block of the stability proteins collagen and elastin. One fourth to one third of the collagen reinforcement rods, for example, are made up of proline. It is easy to understand how important it is for the optimum stability of our blood vessels and our body in general to get an optimum amount of proline in our diet.

Proline is also very important in the process of reversing atherosclerotic deposits. As described in this book in detail, cholesterol-carrying fat globules (lipoproteins) are attached to the inside of the blood vessel wall via biological adhesive tapes. Proline is a formidable "Teflon" agent, which can neutralize the stickiness of these fat globules. The therapeutic effect is two-fold. First, proline helps to prevent the further build-up of atherosclerotic deposits; second, proline helps to release already deposited fat globules from the blood vessel wall into the blood stream. When many fat globules are released from the plaques in the artery walls, the deposit size decreases, leading to a reversal of cardiovascular disease.

Proline can be synthesized by the body, but the amounts synthesized are frequently too little, particularly in patients with an increased risk for cardiovascular disease.

Lysine

As opposed to proline, lysine is an essential amino acid, which means that the body cannot synthesize this amino acid at all. A daily supplementation of this amino acid is therefore critical. Lysine, like proline, is an important building block of collagen and of other stability molecules and its intake helps to stabilize the blood vessels and the other organs in the body.

Lysine is another "Teflon" agent, which can help release deposited fat globules from the blood vessel walls. People with existing cardiovascular disease may increase their daily intake of lysine and proline to several grams in addition to the basic program recommended in this book.

Lysine is also the precursor for the amino acid carnitine. The conversion from lysine into carnitine requires the presence of vitamin C as a biocatalyst. This is another reason why the combination of lysine with vitamin C is essential.

The combined intake of lysine and proline with vitamin C is of particular importance for optimum stability of body tissue. For optimum strength of the collagen molecules, their building blocks lysine and proline need to be modified to hydroxy-lysine and hydroxy-proline. Vitamin C is the most effective biocatalyst to accomplish this "hydroxylation" reaction, thereby providing optimum strength to the connective tissue.

Arginine

Arginine has many functions in the human body. In connection with the cardiovascular system, one function is of particular importance. The amino acid arginine can split off a small molecule called nitric oxide. This tiny part of the former arginine molecule has a powerful role in maintaining cardiovascular health. Nitric oxide relaxes the blood vessel walls and thereby helps to normalize high blood pressure. In addition, nitric oxide helps to decrease the stickiness of platelets and thereby has an anti-clogging effect.

Carnitine

Carnitine is an extremely important amino acid and essential nutrient. It is needed for the proper conversion of fat into energy. Carnitine functions like a shuttle between the cell factory and the energy compartment within each cell. It transports energy molecules in and out of these cellular power plants. This mechanism is particularly important for all muscle cells, including those of the heart. For the constantly pumping heart, carnitine is one of the most critical cell fuels. Thus, it is not surprising that many clinical studies have documented the great value of carnitine supplementation in improving the performance of the heart.

Carnitine also benefits the electrical cells of the heart, and its supplementation has been shown to help normalize different forms of irregular heartbeat.

Cysteine
Cysteine is another important amino acid with many important functions in our body. The cardiovascular system benefits particularly from supplementation with this amino acid because cysteine is a building block of glutathione, one of the most important antioxidants produced in the body. Among others, glutathione protects the inside of the blood vessel walls from free radical and other damage.

OTHER IMPORTANT NUTRIENTS

Coenzyme Q-10
Coenzyme Q-10 is an essential nutrient, also known as ubiquinone. Coenzyme Q-10 functions as an extremely important catalyst for the energy center of each cell.

Because of their high work load, the heart muscle cells have a particularly high demand for Coenzyme Q-10. In patients with insufficient heart pumping function, this essential nutrient is frequently deficient. An irrefutable number of clinical studies have documented the great value of Coenzyme Q-10 in the treatment of heart failure and for optimum heart performance.

Inositol
Inositol is essential for sugar and fat metabolism in the cells of our body.

Inositol is also important for the biological communication process between the cells and organs of our body. Hormones such as insulin, and other molecules, are signals from outside the cell. If a hormone docks to a cell, it wishes to transmit information to this cell. Inositol is part of the proper reading mechanism of this information through the cell membrane. Thus, inositol is part of the proper biological communication process, which, in turn, is critical for optimum cardiovascular health.

Pycnogenols

Pycnogenols refers to a group of bioflavonoids (pro-anthocyanidins) with remarkable properties. In the cardiovascular system, pycnogenols have several important functions:

• Pycnogenols are powerful antioxidants that work together with vitamin C and vitamin E in preventing damage to the cardiovascular system by free radicals.

• Together with vitamin C, pycnogenols have a particular value in stabilizing the blood vessel walls, including the capillaries. Pycnogenols have been shown to bind to elastin, the most important elasticity molecule, and protect elastin molecules against enzymatic degradation.

Biological Targets for Optimal Cardiovascular Health

Conventional Approaches

The use of specific vitamins and essential nutrients stands in comparison to any other preventive cardiovascular approach. Conventional preventive approaches focus on cholesterol-lowering, reduction of other risk factors, and lifestyle changes. Cardiovascular prevention programs based on lifestyle changes alone are limited by the fact that they lack key targets of cardiovascular health such as optimum antioxidant protection, optimum vascular stability and repair, as well as optimum resupplementation of cell fuels.

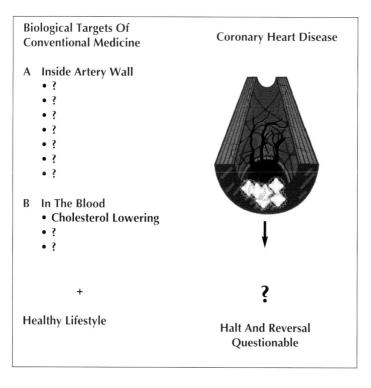

Biological Targets Of Conventional Medicine

Coronary Heart Disease

A   Inside Artery Wall
  - ?
  - ?
  - ?
  - ?
  - ?
  - ?
  - ?

B   In The Blood
  - Cholesterol Lowering
  - ?
  - ?

+

Healthy Lifestyle

?

Halt And Reversal Questionable

Cellular Health

In contrast, the use of vitamins and specific nutrients has defined biological targets. No other currently available preventive health program targets the main problems of cardiovascular disease in such a direct and comprehensive way. Vascular wall stability is optimized. Vascular healing processes are induced. Antioxidant and "Teflon" protection is provided. The most important biological targets of the natural cardiovascular health program are summarized in the figure below.

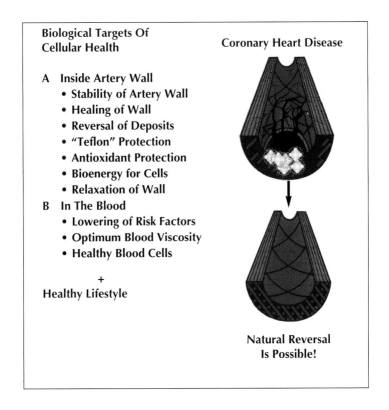

Biological Targets Of Cellular Health

Coronary Heart Disease

A   Inside Artery Wall
  • Stability of Artery Wall
  • Healing of Wall
  • Reversal of Deposits
  • "Teflon" Protection
  • Antioxidant Protection
  • Bioenergy for Cells
  • Relaxation of Wall
B   In The Blood
  • Lowering of Risk Factors
  • Optimum Blood Viscosity
  • Healthy Blood Cells

+
Healthy Lifestyle

Natural Reversal Is Possible!

Vitamin Programs Compared To Conventional Therapies Effectiveness

Conventional therapy is generally limited to the treatment of cardiovascular symptoms one at a time. Since most heart disease patients have many cardiovascular problems at the same time, they frequently are prescribed several medications.

In contrast, vitamin programs correct the underlying causes of the disease. They provide the cell fuels for millions of cells, allowing for correction of impaired cellular function in different compartments of the cardiovascular system at the same time. With this figure I would also like to encourage my colleagues in medicine to use causal therapies wherever possible.

Conventional Medicine Primarily Treats Symptoms

Medication Type	Treatment of Symptoms
Nitrate Group	➤ Angina Pectoris (Symptoms)
Antiarrhythmic Drugs ➤	Arrhythmia (Symptoms)
Betablocker Group	➤ High Blood Pressure (Symptoms)
Diuretic Group	➤ Heart Failure (Symptoms)

Cellular Health Therapy Aims To Correct Underlying Causes

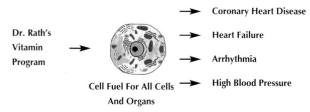

Dr. Rath's Vitamin Program → ➤ Coronary Heart Disease

➤ Heart Failure

➤ Arrhythmia

Cell Fuel For All Cells And Organs → High Blood Pressure

Safety

Another important advantage of vitamin programs compared to conventional drug therapies is that they are safe, and without side effects. Dr. A. Bendich recently summarized the safety aspects of vitamins in a review for the New York Academy of Sciences. She found that all rumors about side effects of vitamins are unsubstantiated.

Apparently, these rumors are only kept alive in the interest of the pharmaceutical industry to scare people and to secure their prescription drug market. In the figure below, the Cellular Health approach is compared with therapies currently offered by conventional medicine. The potential side effects of these conventional drugs are listed with their references.

Conventional Medicine

Therapy	Potential Side Effects	References
Cholesterol-Lowering Drugs	Cancer, Liver Damage Myopathy (Muscle Weakness)	Physician's Desk Reference (PDR)
Aspirin	Strokes, Ulcers, Collagen Breakdown May Actually Promote Heart Disease	PDR Brooks
Calcium-Blocker	Cancer	Psaty

Cellular Health

Therapy	Potential Side Effects	References
Essential Nutrients	None	Bendich,

How You Can Live Longer And Stay Healthy

Your body is as old as your cardiovascular system

The same biological mechanisms that lead to the hardening of arteries and to cardiovascular disease determine the process of aging in your body. One could say that the aging of your body is a slow form of cardiovascular disease. The speed at which it ages is directly dependent on the state of your cardiovascular system. Particularly important is the optimum functioning of the 60,000-mile-long walls of your arteries, veins, and capillaries. This blood vessel pipeline supplies all organs of your body and billions of body cells with oxygen and essential nutrients.

If you do not protect your body with essential nutrients, the aging process leads to a gradual thickening of your blood vessel walls. This eventually leads to malnutrition of billions of your body cells, and to an accelerated aging of your entire body and its organs.

Daily supplementation with vitamins, minerals, amino acids and other essential nutrients is a proven way to protect your cardiovascular system. It is also the best way to help retard the aging process of your body in a natural way, thereby contributing to a long and healthy life.

11

The Path to Eradicating Heart Disease

New Era of Human Health Begins

Principles of a New Health Care System

The Rath-Pauling Manifesto

About the Author

A New Era of Human Health Begins

Five hundred years ago, the Roman Catholic church was making billions of Thaler (early currency) by selling indulgences, an imaginary "key to heaven" to its believers. Then the fraudulent scheme collapsed along with it much of the power of the church. Today, the pharma-business tries to sell the "key to health" to millions of people and takes away billions of dollars in return for an illusion: that the pharmaceutical industry knows the solution to your health.

Considering this state of affairs, the urgency for a new healthcare system is obvious. The liberation from the domination of the pharmaceutical industry will immediately and directly benefit millions of people, the business community and the public sector of all nations. This new healthcare system is based on knowledge, and individual responsibility. Basic health has become understandable, possible and affordable for everyone. The era in human history when health was delegated to an industry that shamelessly exploited it is over and gone.

The new healthcare system focuses on primary care, prevention, and eradication of diseases. Health food stores may evolve into community health centers.

The new healthcare system is being built by dedicated lay people together with a growing number of doctors and health professionals. The majority of health professionals are realizing they have been compromised by pharmaceutical companies and have become victims of a drug-centered healthcare.

Principles of a New Healthcare System

1 **Health is understandable for everyone.** The basic causes of human health and disease are understandable for everyone. The fact that millions of body cells regularly need vitamins and other bioenergy supply can be understood by every child.

2 **Health is possible for everyone.** Cellular Health and the daily supply of vitamins and other bioenergy carriers allow everyone to maintain and restore basic physical health.

3 **Health is safely attainable for everyone.** Nature itself provides us with vitamins and other powerful preventive and therapeutic substances to combat human diseases. They are safe for everyone and without side effects.

4 **Health is affordable for everyone.** Effective health measures to prevent the most common human diseases can be offered in any country of the world at a fraction of today's cost. Implementation of Cellular Health as a health measure immediately liberates trillions of dollars in private and public funds.

5 **Health is a human right.** Having access to optimum health is a basic human right. No pharmaceutical company and no government has the right to limit the spread of information about the benefits of vitamins and other natural therapies. Every country in the world should guarantee access to optimum health to its citizens.

6 **Effective healthcare focuses on prevention.** Future medical research and healthcare will focus on the prevention and eradication of diseases rather than on therapies that merely relieve the symptoms of diseases.

7 **Effective healthcare focuses on primary healthcare.** Community based primary healthcare is the key to effective and affordable health care in any country of the world. Health consultants and health centers in every community will replace an ineffective and expensive focus on high-tech medicine.

8 **Medical research has to be under public control.** Public funds for medical research should be used primarily to develop treatments that prevent and eradicate diseases, rather than on merely relieving symptoms and creating dependencies.

The Rath-Pauling Manifesto

The following document was handwritten by Linus Pauling and signed by him in the names of two scientists, Dr. Pauling and Dr. Rath. With this last public appeal, Linus Pauling supported the scientific breakthrough reported in this book. With this historic document the two-time Nobel Laureate with his own hand passed on the torch of nutritional research to the next generation.

A Call for an International Effort to
Abolish Heart Disease

Heart disease, stroke, and other forms of cardiovascular disease now kill millions of people every year and cause millions more to be disabled. There now exists the opportunity to reduce greatly this Toll of death and disability by the optimum dietary supplementation with vitamins and other essential nutrients.

THE GOAL OF ELIMINATING
HEART DISEASE AS THE
MAJOR CAUSE OF DEATH
AND DISABILITY IS
NOW IN SIGHT!

Matthias Rath and Linus Pauling

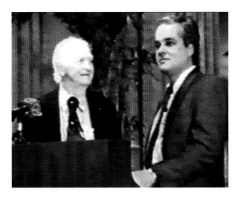

Dr. Pauling and Dr. Rath at the Press Conference in San Francisco on July 2, 1992.

CALL FOR AN INTERNATIONAL EFFORT TO ABOLISH HEART DISEASE

Heart disease, stroke, and other forms of cardiovascular disease now kill millions of people every year and cause millions more to be disabled. There now exists the opportunity to reduce greatly this toll of death and disability by the optimum dietary supplementation with vitamins and other essential nutrients.

During recent years we and our associates have made two remarkable discoveries. One is that the primary cause of heart disease is the insufficient intake of ascorbate (vitamin C), an insufficiency from which nearly every person on earth suffers. Ascorbate deficiency leads to weakness of the walls of the arteries and to the initiation of the atherosclerotic process, particularly in stressed regions. We conclude that cholesterol and other blood risk factors increase the risk for heart disease only if the wall of the artery is weakened by ascorbate deficiency.

The other discovery is that the main cholesterol transporting particle forming atherosclerotic plaques is not LDL (low density lipoprotein) but a related lipoprotein, lipoprotein (a). Moreover, certain essential nutrients, especially the amino acid L-lysine, can block the deposition of this lipoprotein and may even reduce existing plaques. We have concluded that the optimum supplementation of ascorbate and some other nutrients could largely prevent heart disease and stroke and be effective in treating existing disease. Published clinical and epidemiological data support this conclusion.

The goal is now in sight: the abolition of heart disease as the cause of disability and mortality for the present generation and future generations of human beings.

WITH MILLIONS OF LIVES EACH YEAR AT STAKE NO TIME SHOULD BE LOST!

- We call upon our colleagues in science and medicine to join in a vigorous international effort, on the levels of both basic research and clinical studies, to investigate the value of vitamin C and other nutrients in controlling heart disease.
- We call upon the national and international health authorities and other health institutions to support this effort with political and financial measures.
- We call upon every human being to encourage local medical institutions and physicians to take an active part in this process.

THE GOAL OF ELIMINATING HEART DISEASE AS THE MAJOR CAUSE OF DEATH AND DISABILITY IS NOW IN SIGHT!

Matthias Rath and Linus Pauling

About The Author

Matthias Rath, M.D. is a world-renowned physician and scientist who pioneered discoveries related to vitamin C and cardiovascular health. He developed nutritional formulations that help promote and maintain healthy cardiovascular function.* He is the holder of United States Patent Number 5,278,189 for just such a formulation.

Dr. Rath developed the Cellular Health concept that relates healthy structure and function of cells to optimal supply of vitamins and essential nutrients. * Dr. Rath's scientific publications have appeared in prestigious scientific journals including the American Heart Association's *Arteriosclerosis, the Proceedings of the National Academy of Sciences* , and others. Dr. Rath is the founder and head of an international research and development firm.

Until 1992, Dr. Rath was Director of Cardiovascular Research at the Linus Pauling Institute in California and published several landmark scientific publications together with the late Linus Pauling. Dr. Rath's commitment to his scientific findings and promotion of natural health was instrumental in his advocacy for natural health legislation (DSHEA and UN Codex Alimentarius). The details of his work are documented in his latest book Ten Years That Changed The Face of Medicine Forever.

Now Dr. Rath is bringing from Europe the latest scientific advances in natural health to promote a new patient-oriented health care system.

Dr.Rath is the founder of Cellular Health, the new understanding that many of today's most common diseases are facilitated by a deficiency of bioenergy in millions of cells - namely of vitamins and other essential nutrients.

Major portions of the revenues from the sales of Dr. Rath's Cellular Health Formulas are reinvested into further research and clinical studies in natural health. Dr. Rath's Cellular Health Formulas are the first natural health products that are systematically subjected to clinical studies, including double-blind placebo controlled trials.

Dr.Rath's Website www.dr-rath-research.org is one of the world's leading online sources for Cellular Health and natural health science.

References

The following comprehensive list of references is compiled to document the broad support Nutritional and Cellular Health already has. You will find these publications in larger public libraries and in the library of any medical school.

Armstrong VW, Cremer P, Eberle E, et al. (1986) The association between serum Lp(a) concentrations and angiographically assessed coronary atherosclerosis. Dependence on serum LDL-levels. Atherosclerosis 62: 249-257.

Altschul R, Hoffer A, Stephen JD. (1955) Influence of nicotinic acid on serum cholesterol in man. Archives of Biochemistry and Biophysics 54: 558-559.

Aulinskas TH, Van Westhuyzen DR, Coetzee GA. (1983) Ascorbate increases the number of low density lipoprotein receptors in cultured arterial smooth muscle cells. Atherosclerosis 47: 159-171.

Avogaro P, Bon G B, Fusello M. (1983) Effect of pantethine on lipids, lipoproteins and apolipoproteins in man. Current Therapeutic Research 33: 488-493.

Bates CJ, Mandal AR, Cole TJ. (1977) HDL. cholesterol and vitamin-C status. The Lancet II: 611.

Beamish R. (1993) Vitamin E - then and now. Canadian Journal of Cardiology 9: 29-31.

Beisiegel U, Niendorf A, Wolf K, Reblin T, Rath M. (1990) Lipoprotein (a) in the arterial wall. European Heart Journal 11 (Supplement E): 174-183.

Berg K. (1963) A new serum type system in man - the Lp system. Acta Pathologica Scandinavia 59: 369-382.

Blumberg A, Hanck A, Sandner G. (1983) Vitamin nutrition in patients on continuous ambulatory peritoneal dialysis (CAPD). Clinical Nephrology 20: 244-250.

Braunwald E, Hrsg. (1992) Heart Disease – A textbook of cardiovascular medicine. W.B. Saunders & Company, Philadelphia.

Briggs M, Briggs M. (1972) Vitamin C requirements and oral contraceptives. Nature 238: 277.

Carlson LA, Hamsten A, Asplund A. (1989). Pronounced lowering of serum levels of lipoprotein Lp(a) in hyperlipidemic subjects treated with nicotinic acid. Journal of Internal Medicine (England) 226: 271-276.

Cherchi A, Lai C, Angelino F, Trucco G, Caponnetto S, Mereto PE, Rosolen G, Manzoli U, Schiavoni G, Reale A, Romeo F, Rizzon P, Sorgente I, Strano A, Novo S, Immordino R. (1985) International Journal of Clinical Pharmacology, Therapy and Toxicology: 569-572.

Chow CK, Changchit C, Bridges RBI, Rein SR, Humble J, Turk J. (1986) Lower levels of vitamin C and carotenes in plasma of cigarette smokers. Journal of the American College of Nutrition 5: 305-312.

Clemetson CAB. (1989) Vitamin C, Volume I-III. CRC Press Inc., Florida.

Cushing GL, Gaubatz JW, Nave ML, Burdick BJ, Bocan TMA, Guyton JR, Weilbaecher D, DeBakey ME, Lawrie GM, Morrisett JD. (1989) Quantitation and localization of lipoprotein (a) and B in coronary artery bypass vein grafts resected at re-operation. Arteriosclerosis 9: 593-603.

Dahlen GH, Guyton JR, Attar M, Farmer JA, Kautz JA, Gotto AM, Jr. (1986) Association of levels of lipoprotein LP(a), plasma lipids, and other lipoproteins with coronary artery disease documented by angiography. Circulation 74: 758-765.

DeMaio SJ, King SB, Lembo NJ, Roubin GS, Hearn JA, Bhagavan HN, Sgoutas DS. (1992) Vitamin E supplementation, plasma lipids and incidence of restenosis after percutaneous transluminal coronary angioplasty (PTCA). Journal of the American College of Nutrition 11: 68-73.

Dice JF, Daniel CW. (1973) The hypoglycemic effect of ascorbic acid in a juvenile-onset diabetic. International Research Communications System: 1: 41.

Digiesi V. (1992) Mechanism of action of coenzyme Q10 in essential hypertension. Current Therapeutic Research 51: 668-672.

England M. (1992) Magnesium administration and dysrhythmias after cardiac surgery: A placebo-controlled, double-blind randomized trial. Journal of the American Medical Association 268: 2395-2402.

Enstrom JE, Kanim LE, Klein MA. (1992) Vitamin C intake and mortality among a sample of the United States population. Epidemiology 3: 194-202.

Ferrari R, Cucchini, and Visioli O. (1984) The metabolical effects of L-carnitine in angina pectoris. International Journal of Cardiology 5: 213-216.

Folkers K, Yamamura Y (Hrsg.). (1976,1979,1981,1984,1986) Biomedical and clinical aspects of coenzyme Q. Volume 1-5. Elsevier Science Publishers, New York.

Folkers K, Vadhanavikit S, Mortensen SA. (1985) Biochemical rationale and myocardial tissue data on the effective therapy of cardiomyopathy with coenzyme Q10. Proceedings of the National Academy of Sciences USA 82: 901-904.

Folkers K, Langsjoen P, Willis R, Richardson P, Xia LJ, Ye CQ, Tamagawa H. (1990) Lovastatin decreases coenzyme Q-10 levels in humans. Proceedings of the National Academy of Sciences USA 87: 8931-8934.

Gaby SK, Bendich A, Singh VN, Machlin LJ (Hrsg.). (1991) Vitamin intake and health. Marcel Dekker Inc. N.Y.

Gaddi A, Descovich GC, Noseda G, Fragiacomo C, Colombo L, Craveri A, Montanari G, Sirtori CR. (1984) Controlled evaluation of pantethine, a natural hypolipidemic compound, in patients with different forms of hyperlipoproteinemia. Atherosclerosis 5: 73-83.

Galeone F, Scalabrino A, Giuntoli F, Birindelli A, Panigada G, Rossi, Saba P. (1983) The lipid-lowering effect of pantethine in hyperlipidemic patients: a clinical investigation. Current Therapeutic Research 34: 383-390.

Genest J Jr., Jenner JL, McNamara JR, Ordovas JM, Silberman SR, Wilson PWF, Schaefer EJ. (1991) Prevalence of lipoprotein (a) Lp(a) excess in coronary artery disease. American Journal of Cardiology 67: 1039-1045.

Gerster H. (1991) Potential role of beta-carotene in the prevention of cardiovascular disease. International Journal of Vitamin and Nutrition Research 61: 277-291.

Gey KF, Stähelin HB, Puska P and Evans A. (1987) Relationship of plasma level of vitamin C to mortality from ischemic heart disease. 110-123. In: Burns JJ, Rivers JM, Machlin LJ (Hrsg.): Third conference on vitamin C. Annals of the New York Academy of Sciences 498.

Gey KF, Puska P, Jordan P, Moser UK. (1991) Inverse correlation between plasma vitamin E and mortality from ischemic heart disease in cross-cultural epidemiology. American Journal of Clinical Nutrition 53: 326, Supplement.

Ghidini O, Azzurro M, Vita A, Sartori G. (1988) Evaluation of the therapeutic efficacy of L-carnitine in congestive heart failure. International Journal of Clinical Pharmacology, Therapy and Toxicology 26: 217-220.

Ginter E. (1973) Cholesterol: Vitamin C controls its transformation into bile acids. Science 179: 702.

Ginter E. (1978) Marginal vitamin C deficiency, lipid metabolism, and atherosclerosis. Lipid Research 16: 216-220.

Ginter E (1991) Vitamin C deficiency cholesterol metabolism and atherosclerosis. Journal of Orthomolecular Medicine 6: 166-173.

Guraker A, Hoeg JM, Kostner G, Papadopoulos NM, Brewer HB Jr. (1985) Levels of lipoprotein Lp(a) decline with neomycin and niacin treatment. Atherosclerosis 57: 293-301.

Halliwell B, Gutteridge JMC (Hrsg.). (1985) Free radicals in biology and medicine. Oxford University Press, London, New York, Toronto.

Harwood HJ Jr, Greene YJ, Stacpoole PW (1986) Inhibition of human leucocyte 3-hydroxy-3-methylglutaryl coenzyme A reductase activity by ascorbic acid. An effect mediated by the free radical monodehydro-ascorbate. Journal of Biological Chemistry 261: 7127-7135.

Hearn JA, Donohue BC, Ba'albaki H, Douglas JS, King SBIII, Lembo NJ, Roubin JS, Sgoutas DS. (1992) Usefulness of serum lipoprotein (a) as a predictor of restenosis after percutaneous transluminal coronary angioplasty. The American Journal of Cardiology 68: 736-739.

Hennekens, C. See: Rimm EB (1993) and Stampfer (1993).

Hermann WJ JR, Ward K, Faucett J. (1979) The effect of tocopherol on high-density lipoprotein cholesterol. American Journal of Clinical Pathology 72: 848-852.

Hemilä H. (1992) Vitamin C and plasma cholesterol. In: Critical Reviews in Food Science and Nutrition 32 (1): 33-57, CRC Press Inc., Florida.

Hoff HF, Beck GJ, Skibinski CI, Jürgens G, O'Neil J, Kramer J, Lytle B. (1988) Serum Lp(a) level as a predictor of vein graft stenosis after coronary artery bypass surgery in patients. Circulation 77: 1238-1244.

Iseri LT. (1986) Magnesium and cardiac arrhythmias. Magnesium 5: 111-126.

Iseri LT, French JH. (1984) Magnesium: nature's physiologic calcium blocker. American Heart Journal 108: 188-193.

Jacques PF, Hartz SC, McGandy RB, Jacob RA, Russell RM. (1987) Ascorbic acid, HDL, and total plasma cholesterol in the elderly. Journal of the American College of Nutrition 6: 169-174.

Kamikawa T, Kobayashi A, Emaciate T, Hayashi H, Yamazaki N. (1985) Effects of coenzyme Q-10 on exercise tolerance in chronic stable angina pectoris. American Journal of Cardiology 56: 247-251.

Koh ET (1984) Effect of Vitamin C on blood parameters of hypertensive subjects. Oklahoma State Medical Association Journal 77: 177-182.

Korbut R. (1993) Effect of L-arginine on plasminogen-activator inhibitor in hypertensive patients with hypercholesterolemia. New England Journal of Medicine 328 [4]:287-288.

Kostner GM, Avogaro P, Cazzolato G, Marth E, Bittolo-Bon G, Qunici GB. (1981) Lipoprotein Lp(a) and the risk for myocardial infarction. Atherosclerosis 38: 51-61.

Langsjoen PH, Folkers K, Lyson K, Muratsu K, Lyson T, Langsjoen P. (1988) Effective and safe therapy with coenzyme Q10 for cardiomyopathy. Klinische Wochenschrift 66: 583-590.

Langsjoen PH, Folkers K, Lyson K, Muratsu K, Lyson T, Langsjoen P. (1990) Pronounced increase of survival of patients with cardiomyopathy when treated with coenzyme Q10 and conventional therapy. International Journal of Tissue Reactions XIII (3) 163-168.

Lavie CJ. (1992) Marked benefit with sustained-release niacin (vitamin B3) therapy in patients with isolated very low levels of high-density lipoprotein cholesterol and coronary artery disease. The American Journal of Cardiology 69: 1093-1085.

Lawn RM. (1992) Lipoprotein (a) in heart disease. Scientific American. June: 54-60.

Lehr, HA, Frei B, Arfors KE. (1994) Vitamin C prevents cigarette smoke-induced leucocyte aggregation and adhesion to endothelium in vivo. Proceedings of the National Academy of Sciences 91: 7688-7692.

Levine M. (1986) New concepts in the biology and biochemistry of ascorbic acid. New England Journal of Medicine 314: 892-902.

Liu VJ, Abernathy RP. (1982) Chromium and insulin in young subjects with normal glucose tolerance. American Journal of Clinical Nutrition 25: 661-667.

Mann GV, Newton P. (1975) The membrane transport of ascorbic acid. Second Conference on Vitamin C. 243-252. Annals of the New York Academy of Sciences.

Mather HM et al. (1979) Hypomagnesemia in diabetes. Clinical and Chemical Acta 95: 235-242.

McBride PE and Davis JE. (1992) Cholesterol and cost-effectiveness implications for practice, policy, and research. Circulation 85: 1939-1941.

McCarron DA, Morris CD, Henry HJ and Stanton JL. (1984) Blood pressure and nutrient intake in the United States. Science 224: 1392-1398.

McNair P et al. (1978) Hypomagnesemia, a risk factor in diabetic retinopathy. Diabetes 27: 1075-1077.

Miccoli R, Marchetti P, Sampietro T, Benzi L, Tognarelli M, Navalesi R. (1984) Effects of pantethine on lipids and apolipoproteins in hypercholesterolemic diabetic and nondiabetic patients. Current Therapeutic Research 36: 545-549.

Mikami H et al. (1990) Blood pressure response to dietary calcium intervention in humans. American Journal of Hypertension 3: 147-151

Newman TB and Hulley SB (1996) Carcinogenicity of lipid-lowering drugs. Journal of the American Medical Association 275: 55-60.

Niedzwiecki A, Ivanov V. (1994) Direct and extracellular matrix mediated effect of ascorbate on vascular smooth muscle cell proliferation. 24th AAA (Age) and 9th American College of Clinical Gerontology Meeting Washington D.C.

Niendorf A, Rath M, Wolf K, Peters S, Arps H, Beisiegel U, Dietel M. (1990) Morphological detection and quantification of lipoprotein (a) deposition in atheromatous lesions of human aorta and coronary arteries. Virchow's Archives of Pathological Anatomy 417: 105-111.

Nunes GL, Sgoutas DS, Redden RA, Sigman SR, Gravanis MB, King SB, Berk BC. (1995) Combination of Vitamin C and E alters the response to coronary balloon injury in the pig. Arteriosclerosis, Thrombosis and Vascular Biology 15: 156-165.

Opie LH. (1979) Review: Role of carnitine in fatty acid metabolism of normal and ischemic myocardium. American Heart Journal 97: 375-388.

Paolisso G et al. (1993) Pharmacologic doses of vitamin E improve insulin action in healthy subjects and in non-insulin-dependent diabetic patients. American Journal of Clinical Nutrition 57: 650-656.

Paterson JC (1941): Canadian Medical Association Journal 44: 114-120.

Pauling L (1986): How to Live Longer and Feel Better. WH Freeman and Company, New York.

Pfleger R, Scholl F. (1937) Diabetes und vitamin C. Wiener Archiv für Innere Medizin 31: 219-230.

Psaty BM, Heckbert SR, Koepsell TD et. al. (1995) The risk of myocardial infarction associated with antihypertensive drug therapies. Journal of the American Medical Association 274: 620-625.

Rath M, Niendorf A, Reblin T, Dietel M, Krebber HJ, Beisiegel U. (1989) Detection and quantification of lipoprotein (a) in the arterial wall of 107 coronary bypass patients. Arteriosclerosis 9: 579-592.

Rath M, Pauling L. (1990a) Hypothesis: Lipoprotein (a) is a surrogate for ascorbate. Proceedings of the National Academy of Sciences USA 87: 6204-6207.

Rath M, Pauling L (1990b) Immunological evidence for the accumulation of lipoprotein (a) in the atherosclerotic lesion of the hypoascorbemic guinea pig. Proceedings of the National Academy of Sciences USA 87: 9388-9390.

Rath M, Pauling L. (1991a) Solution to the puzzle of human cardiovascular disease: Its primary cause is ascorbate deficiency, leading to the deposition of lipoprotein (a) and fibrinogen/fibrin in the vascular wall. Journal of Orthomolecular Medicine 6: 125-134.

Rath M, Pauling L. (1991b) Apoprotein(a) is an adhesive protein. Journal of Orthomolecular Medicine 6: 139-143.

Rath M., Pauling L. (1992a) A unified theory of human cardiovascular disease leading the way to the abolition of this disease as a cause for human mortality. Journal of Orthomolecular Medicine 7: 5-15.

Rath M, Pauling L. (1992b) Plasmin-induced proteolysis and the role of apoprotein(a), lysine, and synthetic lysine analogs. Journal of Orthomolecular Medicine 7: 17-23.

Rath M. (1992c) Lipoprotein-a reduction by ascorbate. Journal of Orthomolecular Medicine 7: 81-82.

Rath M. (1992d) Solution to the puzzle of human evolution. Journal of Orthomolecular Medicine 7: 73-80.

Rath M. (1992e) Reducing the risk for cardiovascular disease with nutritional supplements. Journal of Orthomolecular Medicine 7: 153-162.

Rath M. (1993c) A new era in medicine. Journal of Orthomolecular Medicine 8: 134-135.

Rath M. (1996) The Process of Eradicating Heart Disease Has Become Irreversible. Journal of Applied Nutrition 48: 22-33.

Rath M., Niedzwiecki A. (1996) Nutritional Supplement Program Halts Progression of Early Coronary Atherosclerosis Documented by Ultrafast Computed Tomography. Journal of Applied Nutrition. 48: 68-78.

Rhoads GG, Dahlen G, Berg K, Morton NE, Dannenberg AL. (1986) Lp(a) Lipoprotein as a risk factor for myocardial infarction. Journal of the American Medical Association 256: 2540-2544.

Riales RR, Albrink MJ. Effect of chromium chloride supplementation on glucose tolerance and serum lipids including high-density lipoprotein of adult men. American Journal of Clinical Nutrition 34: 2670-2678.

Riemersma RA, Wood DA, Macintyre CCA, Elton RA, Gey KF, Oliver MF. (1991) Risk of angina pectoris and plasma concentrations of vitamins A, C, and E and carotene. The Lancet 337: 1-5.

Rimm EB, Stampfer MJ, Ascherio AA, Giovannucci E, Colditz GA, Willett WC. (1993) Vitamin E consumption and the risk of coronary heart disease in men. New England Journal of Medicine 328: 1450-1449.

Rivers JM. (1975) Oral contraceptives and ascorbic acid. American Journal of Clinical Nutrition 28: 550-554.

Rizzon P, Biasco G, Di Biase M, Boscia F, Rizzo U, Minafra F, Bortone A, Silprandi N, Proco-pio A, Bagiella E, Corsi M. (1989) High doses of L-carnitine in acute myocardial infarction: metabolic and antiarrhythmic effects. European Heart Journal 10: 502-508.

Rudolph Willi (1939) Vitamin C und Ernährung. Enke Verlag Stuttgart.

Salonen JT, Salonen R, Ihanainen M, Parviainen M, Seppänen R, Seppänen K, Rauramaa R. (1987) Vitamin C deficiency and low linolenate intake associated with elevated blood pressure: The Kuopio Ischemic Heart Disease Risk Factor Study. Journal of Hypertension 5 (Supplement 5): S521-S524.

Salonen JT, Salonen R, Seppäneen K, Rinta-Kiikka S, Kuukka M, Korpela H, Alfthan G, Kantola M, Schalch W. (1991) Effects of antioxidant supplementation on platelet function: a ran-domized pair-matched, placebo-controlled, double-blind trial in men with low antioxi-dant status. American Journal of Clinical Nutrition 53: 1222-1229.

Sauberlich HE, Machlin LJ (Hrsg.). (1992) Beyond deficiency: new views on the function and health effects of vitamins. Annals of the New York Academy of Sciences 669.

Smith HA, Jones TC, Hrsg. (1958) Veterinary Pathology.

Sokoloff B, Hori M, Saelhof CC, Wrzolek T, Imai T. (1966) Aging, atherosclerosis and ascorbic acid metabolism. Journal of the American Gerontology Society 14: 1239-1260.

Som S, Basu S, Mukherjee D, Deb S, Choudhury PR, Mukherjee S, Chatterjee SN, Chatterjee IB. (1981) Ascorbic acid metabolism in diabetes mellitus. Metabolism 30: 572-577.

Spittle CR. (1971) Atherosclerosis and vitamin C. Lancet ii, 1280-1281.

Stampfer M. et al. (1993) Vitamin E consumption and the risk of coronary heart disease in women. New England Journal of Medicine 328: 1444-1449.

Stankova L, Riddle M, Larned J, Burry K, Menashe D, Hart J, Bigley R. (1984) Plasma ascorbate concentrations and blood cell dehydroascorbate transport in patients with diabetes melli-tus. Metabolism 33: 347-353.

Vital Statistics of the United States, US Department of Health and Human Services, National Center for Health Statistics, 1994.

World Health Statistics, World Health Organization, Genf, 1994.

Stepp W, Schroeder H, Altenburger E. (1935) Vitamin C und Blutzucker. Klinische Wochen-schrift 14 [26]: 933-934.

Stryer L. (1988) Biochemistry. 3rd edition. W.H. Freeman and Company New York.

Tarry WC. (1994) L-arginine improves endothelium-dependent vasorelaxation and reduces initial hyperplasia after balloon angioplasty. Arteriosclerosis and Thrombosis 14: 938-943.

Teo KK, Salim Y. (1993) Role of magnesium in reducing mortality in acute myocardial infarction: A review of the evidence. Drugs 46[3]: 347-359.

Thomsen JH, Shug AL, Yap VU et al. (1979) Improved pacing tolerance of the ischemic human myocardium after administration of carnitine. American Journal of Cardiology 43: 300-306.

Turlapaty PDMV, Altura BM. (1980) Magnesium deficiency produces spasms of coronary arteries: relationship to etiology of sudden death ischemic heart disease. Science 208: 198-200.

Virchow R. (1859) Cellularpathologie. Verlag von August Hirschwald, Berlin.

Widman L et al. (1993) The dose-dependent reduction in blood pressure through administration of magnesium: A double-blind placebo controlled cross-over study. American Journal of Hypertension 6: 41-45.

Willis GC, Light AW, Gow WS. (1954) Serial arteriography in atherosclerosis. Canadian Medical Association Journal 71: 562-568.

Zenker G, Koeltringer P, Bone G, Kiederkorn K, Pfeiffer K, Jürgens G. (1986) Lipoprotein (a) as a Strong Indicator for Cardiovascular Disease. Stroke 17: 942-945.